A PRACTICAL GUIDE TO QUALITATIVE HEALTHCARE

A PRACTICAL GUIDE TO QUALITATIVE HEALTHCARE

Jane Gabbidon

To order additional copies of this book, contact:
Xlibris
1-888-795-4274
www.Xlibris.com
Orders@Xlibris.com
708122

CONTENTS

DEDICATION

To the many professional and para professional health-care providers who have chosen long-term care as their passion and strive every day to provide our residents and their families with the highest quality of care, I salute you. To the residents and their families who have entrusted us with their care we say thank you.

I dedicate this book to the honor and loving memory of my mother, Ann Wade Buffong.

PREFACE

The health care profession is one of the most, if not the most, regulated profession in the USA. It is regulated by the county, the state and at the federal level. Every aspect of care in a health care facility is governed by some form of regulation. Most of these governing regulations are not taught in schools and are only introduced to health care clinicians, professionals as well as the para-professionals by health care delivery institutions. However, it is the effective implementation of these regulations in the health care industry that translates to successful patient outcomes and the delivery of quality healthcare to the community. Health care Providers deviation from the state and federal regulations is most often not a deliberate attempt to be non-compliant but rather a lack of knowledge as to what the regulations are.

This book was designed as an interpretation of the state and federal regulations in conjunction with many best practices to familiarize all healthcare professionals and para professionals of the state and federal regulations that affect health care delivery.

Nursing homes, hospitals, assisted living communities, adult homes, group homes and anyone considering employment in the health care industry will all benefit from the contents of this book.

Residents, families and friends of residents will also benefit from the contents of this book in two ways (a). It informs them of their rights and (b) they will enjoy good quality care when the providers follow the regulations.

FOREWORD

Like a community, every health care facility is made up of different departments. No single person is the master of health care delivery. It is a collaborative interdisciplinary effort. On a daily basis, our health care system operates on a reversed pyramid. The insight of the para professions who are the direct care givers and interaction with our residents more frequently are often the driving force behind the immediate care provided by the professionals. The goal of each health care facility provider is to provide quality health care that is in alignment with the regulations. However, too often there is a lack of knowledge of what the regulations are as these are only introduced to the health-care employee upon entry into the health-care industry.

This author adds energy, personal experience, and color to what in other publications can be a rather boring tale of the concepts and practices of our healthcare system. She adequately outlines most, if not all, of the areas that a newly graduated or experienced health care professional can use to assist him or her navigate our complex health-care system.

There are "how to do it" books but very few, if any, that cover all the elements as is the case here. It can be read as how policy and regulations are translated into practice with the lessons learned from experience. This book is a guide that many healthcare staff, especially those in long term care, can relate to and use in their everyday working life as a guide to attain and maintain the best patient outcomes.

David Roberts, RN Consultant
Chief Nursing Officer
Medical Director Services

APPRECIATION

I would like to thank my colleagues whose suggestions made this a better book than it would otherwise have been. Working with you has made the creation of this book a stimulating and gratifying experience. I cannot mention everybody's name, but I most especially thank the following people: Lenox Carroll, RN Assistant Director of Nursing; Helen Okonkwo, RNC, BSN, MS-HSMG, Director of Nursing/ Regional Nurse Consultant; AnnMarie Akinyooye, RN, Director of Nursing; Edwine Joseph, RN, Director of Nursing.

To the many other colleagues not mentioned but were happy to answer a question along the way or review a chapter, Thank you. To the Administrators, Medical Directors, Doctors, Nurses, MDS Coordinators, Certified Nursing Assistants, Social Workers, Dietitians, Rehabilitation staff, Recreation Staff, Food Service Directors, Dietary Staff, Maintenance staff, Housekeeping staff, Finance office personal, Admissions personnel all consultants and non-medical colleagues, Thank You.

I would also like to say a special thank you to my uncle, Mr. James Wade who always encourage me to never limit my possibilities.

SCOPE AND SEVERITY OF
CITATIONS DURING SURVEY

Every healthcare facility is surveyed either by the state or by the federal government within 10 to 12 months following the previous survey. It is the government's way of ensuring that these facilities are operating in accordance with the regulations governing that facility and that residents are receiving quality care. At the end of the survey, facilities are informed of issues identified and these are referred to as citations or tags. A formal written report will then be issued by the state.

1. Survey citations or tags in nursing homes, as outlined throughout this book, are F tags.
2. The tags have a number assigned to them for identification purposes. E.g. F309, F157 etc.
3. There are also K tags, which are environmental issues, safety issues, and fire codes.
4. Although K tags mostly relate to environmental issues, they can at times also be cited for clinically related issues. E.g. room temperatures and resident comfort and safety issues.
5. When a facility is cited for deficient practice, it is an F tag, as outlined throughout this book. However, what holds equal or more weight is the scope and severity of that F tag.
6. Scope and severity is a system of rating the seriousness of deficiencies. It is a national system used by all state survey agencies when conducting nursing home Medicare and Medicaid certification surveys.
7. For each deficiency identified, the surveyor determines the level of harm to the resident (s) involved (severity) and the scope of the problem within the nursing home.
8. The surveyor then assigns an alphabetical scope and severity value from A through L with "A" being the least serious and "L" the most serious.
9. The letters "J' 'K' and "L" for any of the regulations is immediate jeopardy.

10. Immediate jeopardy is a situation in which the facility's non-compliance with one or more of regulations has place resident (s) at risk for abuse, harm, injury, impairment or death or <u>potential for harm.</u>
11. Immediate jeopardy can be an isolated incident or widespread.
12. When the survey results or Statement of Deficiency (SOD) are received from the state, the facility has ten business days to prepare and send back a plan of correction (POC). In New York State, this can be monitored on the Health Commerce System (HCS).
13. Upon submission of the plan of correction (POC), the facility must receive notice from the state whether the POC was accepted or if changes are required.
14. If the facility disagrees with a particular tag, it can file an Informal Dispute Resolution (IDR), which allows the facility to provide additional information that may result in revision and/or reversal of the statement of deficiency.
15. The State always conduct a post survey revisit after every plan of correction is submitted. This revisit is often done as a follow-up phone call to ensure the facility is in compliance with the stated plan of correction.
16. When a facility receives a level **<u>G</u>** or an **<u>Immediate Jeopardy (IJ)</u>** tag, the post survey revisit involves an actual onsite revisit by the State within ninety days to validate correction of deficiencies.
17. **NOTE:** As part of the preparation for survey of a facility, the survey team looks at a four year history of a facility's deficiencies from past surveys and complaint surveys. During the survey, they will check to see if there are repeat deficiencies!
18. The following chart is an abbreviated version of how scope is determined.

	Scope of the Deficiency		
Severity of the Deficiency	Isolated	Pattern	Widespread
Immediate jeopardy to resident health or safety	J	K	L

Actual harm that is not immediate jeopardy	G	H	I
No actual harm with potential for more than minimal harm that is not immediate jeopardy	D	E	F
No actual harm with potential for minimal harm	A	B	C

Shaded boxes in the grid mean deficiency ratings which reflect Substandard Quality of Care. These areas are mainly:

Physical or chemical restraints
Abuse not addressed
Staff mistreatment of residents-verbal, mental, physical or sexual abuse

Employing individuals who have been found guilty of abuse, neglect or mistreatment
Dignity issues
Lack of resident choices
Preventing resident from organizing or participating in a group in or out of facility
Not providing notice before room or roommate change.
Lack of adequate activities and a qualified activities director
Not making sure residents have adaptive equipment and these are properly applied
Misplacement of residents' clothing and personal items
Failure to notification family of changes to residents' plan of care
Lack of discharge planning and follow-up
Lack of consultation services
Pain not properly addressed
Not having a qualified social worker who addresses residents needs and individuality
Environment is not safe, clean, comfortable and homelike

Poor housekeeping and laundry practices
Uncomfortable temperatures and sounds
Residents decline and not properly accessed and care planned
Lack of qualified nursing staff
Lack of a Medical Director
Development of pressure ulcers not properly documented
Inadequate care of hospice residents
Inadequate care of dialysis residents

For each letter of deficiency received, the state has different categories of penalty that it can be imposed on facilities.

1. Category 1—Directed Plan of Correction (obtain services of an outside consultant)
   --Directed In-service training (comprehensive outline for in-services)

2. Category 2—Denial of payment for new admissions
   --Denial of payments for all residents
   --Civil Money Penalties of $50.00 to $3,000.00 per day

3. Category 3—Temporary Management
   --Immediate Termination
   --Civil Money Penalties of $3,050 to $10,000 per day.

ADMISSION OF A RESIDENT

Before admitting an individual to a long term care skilled facility, the facility must thoroughly review the submitted documentation and ensure it can meet the needs of that individual. Hospitals, acute care setting, group homes, adult homes or home settings must complete and submit documentation to the long term care facility for review to determine the needs of the individual prior to consent for admission.

In New York State the required documentations are a PRI (Patient Review Instrument) and a Screen. The combination of both documents is referred to as a Level 1 PASRR (Pre-Admission Screening and Resident Review).

NOTE: A PRI alone is not complaint with the PASRR regulation! Must receive the PRI and the Screen!

These documents are completed by the referring institution by a health care professional who has completed the State's PRI and Screen certification course and have been issued a PRI and a Screen identification number.

The PRI (Patient Review Instrument) is a medical tool that identifies whether or not a resident is qualified for skilled nursing care. The PRI provides demographic information including the payer source, diagnoses, level of care required with activities of daily living such as eating, transferring from one surface to another, toileting needs, need for therapy, current medications individual is receiving, an outline of the care and services received prior to admission to the long term care setting, need for follow-up consultations and the individual's preferred living arrangements.

The Screen is a document that determines if there is a substantial medical need to require admission to a long term care setting rather than medical services that can be easily given in the community. If the completed Screen indicates that the individual has Mental Illness, Mental Retardation or Developmental Disabilities, the resident then requires a level 2 PASRR (Pre-Admission Screening and Resident Review).

There are two agencies responsible for level 2 PSARR completion:

1. Individuals with <u>Mental Illness</u> require a level 2 PSARR which is done by a government appointed regulatory agency which in New York State is IPRO (Island Peer Review Organization). These trained Mental Health Professions review and make the determination on whether an individual with <u>Mental Illness</u> can be admitted to a long term care setting.
2. Individuals with <u>Mental Retardation and Developmental Disabilities</u> require a level 2 PSARR which is done by New York State Developmental Disabilities Service Office.

An individual with Mental Illness, Mental Retardation and Developmental Disabilities can only be admitted to a long term care skilled facility if approved by the aforementioned.

NOTE: Failure to comply with this process is a violation of the Federal PSARR regulation and can result in as much as Immediate Jeopardy!

NOTE: Each time a resident requires hospitalization, a new PRI and screen must be submitted to the skilled care facility prior to re-admission.

NOTE: Surveyors generally ask for the level 1 PASRR (PRI and Screen) for all residents been reviewed and a list of residents with level 2 PSARR to ascertain if residents with Mental Illness, Mental Retardation or Developmental Disabilities are appropriately placed in a long term care facility!

NOTE: Upon admission, Social Services MUST review all level 1 and level 2 PSARRS.

NOTE: It is advisable for them to copy the PSARR and keep a copy in their section of the medical records and a list of ALL residents who are level 2 PSARR.

NOTE: Social Services documentation on all residents should clearly reflect ongoing need for continued admission, especially residents with level 2 PSARR.

For all admissions, a thorough review of submitted documentation must be conducted to ensure the facility can meet the individual's needs to minimize re-hospitalization. E.g. approving a level 1 PASRR for a ventilator resident when the facility does not have a ventilator unit. E.g. approving a resident with a positive level 2 PSARR without the accompanying clearance from the regulatory agency.

Potential tag: F285—PSARR Requirement for Mental Illness and Mental Retardation

ASSESSMENT OF A RESIDENT

When a resident is admitted to a skilled care facility, a thorough head to toe assessment must be done and the resident must be made aware of his or her rights. Assessment and discharge start on admission and are ongoing. An initial full clinical assessment is done but throughout the course of the resident's stay in the facility, there is ongoing assessment by the interdisciplinary team to ensure that the resident is receiving the highest level of care needed to attain and maintain his or her physical, mental and psychological well being in accordance with the regulations. These areas include but are not limited to:

Residents aware of their rights to quality of life and to receive necessary care in a dignified manner
Minimum Data Set (MDS)
Care Planning
Pain or discomfort management
Wound treatment and prevention
Prevention of medication errors either by the delivery system or storage system
Accident/Incident prevention
Potential for elopement properly assessed and resident safety ensured
Prevention of abuse, neglect and mistreatment and ensured follow-up in suspected cases
Care for by staff with no criminal backgrounds
Adequate staff to ensure residents needs are met
Staff members are trained and competent to take care of their needs
Free from physical restraints
Assessment of why resident is refusing care/treatments
Right to refuse or to implement advance directives
Physician Services including choice of a physician
Medical care supervised by a Medical Director
Aware of the facility's discharge, transfer and bed hold policy
Resident/family right to notification of any changes to the Resident's plan of care

Right to be free from misappropriation of personal property
Enjoy meaningful therapeutic recreation
The right to smoke
Dietary needs including weight management
Dining Observation
Sanitary food storage, preparation and distribution
Management of nasogastric or gastrostomy tubes
Receives appropriate consistency foods and liquids
Fluid restrictions monitoring if required
Residents with special needs e.g. dialysis, indwelling catheters, colostomy, ileostomy, oxygen usage, blood glucose monitoring
Treatment and Prevention of Infections
Immunizations
Receive all Necessary Consults
Receive all necessary labs and x-rays
Dental services
Hearing Aid and Eyeglasses
Need for Rehabilitation Services
Maintain at optimal functional level without any decline
Ongoing maintenance of a clean, sanitary home-like environment
Appropriate noise levels
A hazard free environment with preparations in the event of an emergency
Ongoing quality assurance programs to review potential for deficient practices
Ensure their private medical records are secure
Prevention of unnecessary hospitalization
Dignified treatment in the event of death

RESIDENTS RIGHTS

Violation of resident's rights, abuse, neglect and mistreatment are the underlying component to most cases reported to the Department of Health!

As per the State Operation Manual, residents in a healthcare facility have the right to autonomy and choice about how they wish to live their everyday lives and received care subjected to the rules of the facility and not in violation of any of the regulatory requirements.

As per the Long Term Care Survey Guide, the following is a list of residents' rights:

1. Residents have the right to vote and to exercise their free rights subject to the facility's rule.(**F151**—Exercise right to vote/Free of Coercion)
2. Facility must honor resident's or legal representative wishes regarding the resident's care (**F152**—Rights exercised by surrogate)
3. Residents and their designated representatives have the right to view their chart and to purchase copies of the medical records. If resident and/or family request to view the chart, it is advisable for this to be supervised to ensure that no documents are removed from the chart. (**F153**—right to access/purchase copies of records)
4. The resident or legal representative have the right to be fully informed of all his/her medical conditions in a language they understand (**F154**—informed of health status/medical condition)
5. Resident has the right to refuse treatments or formulate advance directives (**155**-Rights to refuse treatments)
6. Resident has the right to be fully informed of the facility's rules, access to the State hotline number and the ombudsman,

access to their doctor and any changes in the facility such as construction (**F156**-inform of services/changes)

7. Residents and/or their family/legal representative must be notified of all changes to the resident or the Resident's plan of care, transfers, discharges, room change or change of roommate. It must be documented they were informed of room/roommate change and agreed to same. (**F157**—notify of significant changes, new wounds, accidents, transfers etc.)

8. The resident has the right to manage their own financial affairs and are not required to deposit their money with the facility (**F158**—resident manage own financial affairs). (However, encourage banking with the facility for safe keeping).

9. Residents *must* have access to their funds seven days a week. Therefore, facility must have a system in place for the hours when the financial office is closed, to ensure residents have access to their funds. MAKE SURE IT IS CLEARLY POSTED IN HIGHLY VISIBLE AREAS HOW MONEY CAN BE OBTAINED WHEN THE BUSINESS OFFICE IS CLOSED. (**F159**—Facility Management of Resident Funds)

10. When a resident is discharged, transferred to another facility, or expires, facility must have a clear, precise policy on allotting resident funds within 30 days. (**F160**—conveyance of personal funds upon death)

11. The facility must safeguard the resident' funds and will reimburse the resident for losses that were the fault of the facility. (**F161**—Surety Bond or other assurance)

12. The facility cannot charge resident for any services for which payment is made by Medicare or Medicaid (**F162**-limitation on charges to personal accounts). Items than can be charged are telephone, television, cigarettes, personal social events and gifts; personal clothing

13. The right to choose or change a physician (**F163**—free choice of personal physician)

14. Resident's record must be kept private and confidential (**F164**—privacy and confidentiality)

15. A resident has the right to voice their dissatisfaction about their care without reprisal (**F165**—voice grievance without reprisal)

16. Resident has the right to be informed of the progress of their grievance regarding their care, funds, lost clothing or violation of their rights. (**F166**—facility resolves resident grievances)
17. Residents and family should have full access to the survey results. These should be placed in a highly visible and accessible area and clearly marked as such. (**F167**—rights to survey results: readily accessible and **168**—Receipt of Info)
18. Resident can perform compensated services for the facility if agreed upon by both parties (**F169**--right to work)
19. Residents have the right to send and receive their mail unopened. Mail should only be opened upon their request and in their presence. (**F170**—right to privacy: send/receive unopened mail)
20. Facility must make sure the resident has access to stationery, pens, and postage. ((**F171**—access to stationery, postage, pens, etc.)
21. Facility cannot block the state or any other government agencies from visiting and speaking with residents. Residents are allowed to have visits from family and friends but with reasonable restrictions imposed by the facility that respects and protects the rights of the resident and other residents. (**F172**—access and visitation)
22. Ombudsman must be granted access to resident's records with the permission of resident or legal representative. (**F173**—Ombudsman access to clinical records)
23. Residents must have access to a telephone and be able to make calls privately. (**F174**—right to telephone access with privacy).
24. Married couples in a facility have the right to share a room. (**F175**—right of married couple to share a room)
25. A resident has the right to self-administer some medications that are deemed safe (e.g., inhalers). However, facility must have protocol in place to ensure that resident
    a. is alert and oriented x3 (Place, Person and Time)
    b. is able to follow directions clearly with return demonstration,
    c. understands the purpose for the medication and potential side effects,
    d. Care plan is completed
    e. Clear indication for ongoing assessment and teaching, and

    f.   Medication written on the medication administration record, which indicates that resident is self-administering but nurse must monitor. (**F176**—resident self-administers drugs if deemed safe)
26. Resident has the right to refuse transfer to another room for billing purposes only (**F177**—Refusal of certain transfers.)

NOTE: The facility CAN discharge a resident if:

Resident refuses to pay for stay at the facility
Health of others is been compromised
Safety of others is endangered
Resident's health has improved and no longer requires services from the facility
Services are necessary to meet resident's welfare which cannot be met in the facility

QUALITY OF LIFE AND DIGNITY

Citations for quality of life and dignity reflect substandard care by a facility!

Every effort must be made by a facility to ensure the residents are treated with dignity and respect and not dehumanized in any way. Some of these areas as per the Long Term Care Guide are:

1. Grooming residents as they wish to be groomed. (E.g. The way they want their hair combed and styled).
2. Encourage residents to be dressed in their own clothing, NOT sitting around in hospital gowns all day. For residents that have no clothing and no involved family, the facility is responsible for ensuring some system of obtaining clothing for them.
3. Transporting residents to activities of their choice.
4. Labelling their clothing in a dignified manner, i.e. label is not visible. (Must take inventory before labelling!)
5. No daily usage of plastic cutlery and no daily usage of paper or plastic plates.
6. Properly covering their clothing at mealtimes with bibs instead of napkins unless this is resident's preference.
7. While providing care to residents, staff should be conversing with the resident NOT with each other.
8. STAFF SHOULD NOT BE STANDING OVER RESIDENTS WHEN FEEDING THEM!
9. Residents' privacy must be respected. Knock on their doors and wait to be invited in. Do not change their TV or radio without their permission. Do not remove or inspect their personal property.
10. **Speaking to residents in a respectful manner.** Address them by the name of THEIR choice. Do not label them. E.g. referring to resident as a feeder.

11. Resident should not be excluded from conversation during group or individual sessions. Do not discuss resident's care in a public forum.
12. Not posting any lists with residents' information that can be read by other residents and visitors. E.g. list of smokers, list of feeders etc.
13. Ensuring resident is well groomed daily and nails trimmed and neat and ensuring that there are no odors.
14. Ensure resident is properly covered to maintain their privacy and dignity. E.g. when taking resident to the shower room, resident should be properly covered, preferable in their own clothing.
15. Foley bags MUST be covered. GT, colostomy, suprapubic should be properly covered for resident's dignity.
16. Residents cannot be refused toileting assistance during meal times.
17. **NOTE:** Residents have the right to be in common spaces such as the lobby if safety is not compromised!
18. Resident should be able to see him/herself in a mirror and have toiletry articles accessible when using the sink.
19. Room can be adjusted if possible to accommodate resident's independence. E.g. there are instances that beds are placed against the wall to allow a wheelchair to maneuver around the room. Any adjustments need to be care planned for!
20. Residents with glasses, hearing aids, dentures should have them in use unless they refuse. Refusals must be documented and interventions must be generated.
21. Resident and family must receive notice before a room or roommate change.

Potential F tag: F240—Care and Environment Promote Quality of Life

Potential F tag F241—Dignity and Respect of Individuality

Potential F tag F246-- Reasonable Accommodation of Needs and Preferences

MDS (MINIMUM DATA SET) COMPLETION

Minimum Data Set (MDS) is a system of providing extensive information on each resident to the State. It provides information on the resident's cognitive status, communication, vision, mood and behavior, level of care required, rehabilitative services needed, continence, diagnoses, dental and nutritional status, skin conditions, accidents/incidents, activities involved in, medications, special treatments/procedures, discharge potential.

Prospective payment system (PPS) is the Medicare payment system. Medicare residents must have MDS completed as follows:

Day 5

Day 14

Day 30

Day 60

Day 90

These are completed as long as the resident remains in the facility and requires a skilled medical or rehabilitative need for that time.

Medicare residents are given one hundred covered days in a nursing home as long as they are skilled. (Copay may apply after day 20). After the resident completes skilled Medicare coverage, if the resident is remaining in the facility, the schedule for MDS completion would be every 92 days, annually or with any significant change and the payer source will change from Medicare to Medicaid (depends on qualification) or resident's other available payer source.

Omnibus Budget Reconciliation Action (OBRA) is the system that regulates Medicaid and other payer sources. These residents must have MDS completed by:

Day 14

Every 92 days

Annually by day 366

Or if there is a significant change to the resident

NOTE: Facilities with paper records, must have a minimum of 15 months of MDS information on the chart. All MDS information is readily accessible on electronic medical records.

Potential tag F272—Comprehensive Assessment

Potential tag: F273—New Admit Comprehensive Assessment

Potential tag: F274—Significant Change Comprehensive Assessment

Potential tag: F275—Yearly Comprehensive Assessment

Potential tag: F276—Quarterly Assessment

F286—Maintain 15 Months of Residents Assessments

CARE PLANNING

The care plan is an interdisciplinary document that addresses all aspects of the resident's care based on a thorough assessment as outlined above. The purpose for care planning is to ensure that all of a Resident's psychological, physical and healthcare needs are identified and met in a timely manner.

1. **ALL** residents when admitted must have an initial care plan started on admission and completed by day 14 and a comprehensive care plan meeting by day 21.
2. Residents and family/legal representatives must be a part of the care planning process.
3. The purpose for a care plan meeting is to meet with the resident and family to review all areas of the comprehensive assessment and plans to meet resident's needs, continuation of the comprehensive assessment by resident and family input and to address any concerns from the resident or family.
4. Social service department must have a clear log that shows that invites are sent out for each care plan meeting and must also show the documentation of responses received. It is advisable to document in the log that notice was sent and document the response in the post care plan wrap up note.
5. The care plan must be updated for every episodic change to the resident's care and with the quarterly assessment every 92 days.
6. A new care plan should be done with the annual assessment.
7. For significant changes, the existing care plan can be updated or a new one written.
8. The care plan must be signed by the interdisciplinary team including the resident and family/legal representative if present at the meeting.
9. If the resident has a wound or history of falls, the old care plan should be stapled to the current to maintain the history. In electronic medical records, the history is maintained.

10. Care plan must be a true accurate description of the resident's needs. E.g. if the resident is exhibiting behavior as simple as repeatedly picking the nose document it on the behavior care plan. It the event of a nose bleed, this may be the root cause. There is no "normal" behavior.
11. Any changes made to a resident's plan of care or to the environment for a resident must be clinically justified on the care plan. E.g. Resident's bed is placed against the wall so that he/she can maneuver wheelchair around. E.g. Resident is provided with a low positioned bed secondary to multiple falls from bed. The justification may be to prevent falls or to minimize injury from falls.
12. It is advisable for the facility to have a system to ensure care plans are updated with every episodic event.
13. Nurses should be taught that every acute change needs to be entered on the care plan promptly to ensure the plan of care remains current.

NOTE: The care plan is only effective when it is correctly implemented. Therefore, interventions written on the care plan **MUST** be shared with the necessary staff. E.g. providing a bed alarm or floor mats after a fall MUST be on the certified nursing assistant accountability record as they are the ones applying these daily. E.g. A resident who has a diagnosis of PICA (eats non-food items such as cigarettes, gloves, etc) MUST be clearly documented on all pertinent records so ALL staff is aware!

NOTE: Care plan meetings can be done via telephone conference per family request!

Potential tag: F279—Develop Comprehensive Care Plan
Potential tag: F280—Resident/Legal Representative Right to Participate in Care Planning And Care Plan Must be revised

PAIN MANAGEMENT

. It is important to recognize, properly assess and treat pain as pain affects mood, appetite, sleep and mobility.

. Expressions of pain may be verbal or nonverbal. Pain threshold varies from individual to individual. Therefore, when the resident requests pain medication, don't be judgmental.

.Pain is subjective and so is the response, including facial expressions, grimacing, groaning, moaning, crying, behavioral changes, screaming, calling out, tendering a specific body part, changes in gait, changes in vital signs, loss of appetite or refusal of care, especially turning and positioning.

. We do have residents who are drug seeking, but is "pain in the mind" different from the resident who has phantom pain on his leg that was amputated months ago?

. It is not the duty of the nurse to be judgmental and withhold or prolong giving a resident pain medications when resident need or request it. This will be considered *abuse* or *mistreatment*. The nurse should provide the pain medications as ordered and notify the doctor of his or her concerns.

. The same also applies for the doctor. If the doctor feels resident is drug seeking, it is advisable to refer him or her to pain management clinic.

.It is advisable for the pain management consultant to have a clear schedule of *all* other medications the resident is on.

. If the attending doctor disagrees with the pain management consultant, that is okay, but it must be clearly documented in the progress notes why he/she is not honoring these recommendations.

. Facility must have an ample emergency supply of pain medication. When pain medication is ordered, it must be given promptly. If the ordered medication is not readily available, the doctor must be notified so that a substitute order that is readily available can be given.

. All residents on pain medications must have a pain scale on the medication administration record to address the severity of pain before and after medication is given.

. Residents should *not* have two as needed (prn) pain medications on the same schedule or close schedules that can result in overdose. (E.g., resident has Tylenol and Motrin ordered for every six hours prn. Who makes the decision as to which one should be given, or should both be given? This is *not* a nurse's decision, so doctor must assess to discontinue one of these medications or give specific instructions as to which one should be given.)

. If a resident has a standing order for pain medication and an as needed order that follows the same time schedule, the doctor needs to state how long after the standing order has been given must the nurse wait to give the as needed medication.

. When as needed pain medications are given, nurses *must* document on the back of the medication administration record why the pain medication was given and whether it was effective; must specify where the resident has pain.

NOTE: If a resident is confused or demented, pain medication should be a standing order, not as needed!

. **NOTE:** If a resident who is demented or confused is agitated, restless, cries or calls out, the doctor should consider putting him/her on a standing order for pain medication as that resident may be in pain but unable to verbalize it and it is not manifested in the usual forms of grimacing, groaning, moaning and or crying etc.!

. Residents on certain pain medications must be monitored for any adverse effects (e.g., constipation or potential for fall).

. Any new onset of pain requires a full assessment to rule out underlying pathology, such as a fracture or other types of injury.

. A pain assessment must be completed on admission, quarterly, annually, with any significant change and with any new onset of pain.

. Nurses should note that certain conditions cause pain and should assess residents with the following conditions for pain meds:

    (a) Pressure ulcers
    (b) Neuropathy
    (c) Stroke
    (d) Amputations (including phantom pain).
    (e) Arthritic changes and contractures
    (f) Status-post surgery
    (g) S/p fall with injuries; fractures, sprains, skin tears, hematomas etc.

. Residents with pain should also be screened by rehab department as sometimes resident may need an ice pack or heat to an area, which is just as effective as pain medications.

. For residents on Tylenol, make sure the daily dosage is not greater than 3grams. This includes combination products like Tylenol with codeine.

. Residents with intractable or difficult to manage pain should be referred to a physiatrist and/or pain clinic.

. MDS must be accurately completed.

.Care plan must be completed.

Potential tag: F272—Comprehensive Assessment
Potential tag: F279—Develop Comprehensive Care Plan
Potential tag: F280—Revision of the Comprehensive Care Plan
Potential tag: F281—Services Provided Meets Professional Standards of Quality Care
Potential tag: F282—Care is provided by a Qualified Person

Potential tag: F309—Provide Care/Services for Highest Well being
Potential tag: F385—Supervision by a Physician
Potential tag: F501—Responsibilities of the Medical Director
Potential tag: 514—Clinical Records Must Reflect Care/Services provided and Response

TRANSDERMAL MEDICATIONS

Transdermal patches are medications that are administered through the skin through a delayed release process. The most frequently used ones are Duragesic, Bengay, Nitroglycerine, Exelon and Nicotine. Duragesic patch is a pain medication and a narcotic and must be stored and treated like all other narcotics. However, all of these patches like all other medications, if not administered properly have an inherent potential for harm.

. Must have doctors order for strength, frequency and how often to apply.

. Documentation must reflect the following:

    a.   Site where it is applied
    b.   How often it is to be applied

. It is advisable to apply patches on hairless areas of the upper back or chest so they are easily located by all nurses.

. Nurses must be mindful to always double check to make sure all old patches are removed before placing a new one.

. Nurse must check for patch placement and sign for patch every shift on the medication administration record.

. Duragesic patch is a narcotic and two nurses must be present for removal and discarding of the patch.

. .Duragesic patch must be discarded in the sharps container (or other non-retrievable place, based on facility policy)

. MDS must clearly reflect medication accordingly.

. Care plan must be completed.

NOTE: If the resident is scheduled for an MRI, remember the patch can cause burns so follow-up with doctor for orders regarding removal and application of a new one upon completion of the procedure.

NOTE: If a resident inadvertently have a new patch placed without removal of the old one, ALL nurses who have signed the medication administration record from application of the second patch until discovery of the medication error are responsible!

Potential tag: F279—Develop Comprehensive Care Plan
Potential tag: F280—Revision of the Comprehensive Care Plan
Potential tag: F281—Services Provided Meets Professional Standards of Quality Care
Potential tag: F282—Care is provided by a Qualified Person
Potential tag—F333—Residents are Free of Significant Medication Errors

PRESSURE ULCERS AND OTHER WOUNDS

Pressure ulcers and other wounds start as an impairment to the skin and can spread to the tissues underlying the skin and can even destroy muscle and bone. Ulcers can be very painful and severely impact on a resident's quality of life. Ulcers can also become infected and lead to systemic complications such as septicemia.

In an attempt to prevent ulcer development, there must is be ongoing monitoring of pressure relief, nutritional status, weight management, incontinence care or other significant decline in a resident' status.

. When a resident is admitted, nurses should be mindful to do a full body assessment with careful attention to often missed areas such as behind the ears, under the breasts, under the armpits, abdominal folds if present, between the buttocks and with emphasis on the feet.

.When a resident is admitted with or develops an ulcer, it must first be determined whether it is a pressure, vascular or diabetic ulcer. If it is determined that it is a pressure ulcer, it must be properly staged. If resident develops a nosocomial (in house) ulcer, it must also be identified as avoidable or unavoidable. A pressure ulcer risk assessment must be done

    a.   on admission or readmission
    b.   with development of any new wounds.
    c.   whenever a new MDS is completed
    d.   with worsening of wounds

. All residents with ulcers must be assessed by the interdisciplinary team:

    a). Doctor must order appropriate treatment and establish baseline pre-albumin levels, supplements such as Vitamin C and Multiple Vitamins and follow up as needed.

b). Rehab department assess for wheelchair cushions, application or removal of devices.

c). Dietary department to ensure adequate caloric intake, and the need for supplements such as Ensure.

d). Social service to ensure the family was notified by the doctor or nursing

. An accident/incident report and investigation should be completed for all new nosocomial (in house) pressure ulcers and other wounds to rule out abuse, neglect or mistreatment and whether an ulcer is avoidable or unavoidable.

. It is preferable to have a wound flow sheet that you can document a weekly note on the back or write a weekly nursing progress note in the resident's chart. (Most electronic medical records allows for a description).

. All wound flow sheets must reflect the following weekly

a. Size (length x width x depth)
b. Location
c. Site
d. *Stage*
e. Place of origin (community or nosocomial)
f. Date originated (for community acquired, should read On Admission))
g. Type of ulcer (pressure, vascular or diabetic)
h. Description of tissue type, i.e. necrotic, denuded, macerated, slough, etc.
i. Drainage if applicable

. If you miss any of the aforementioned, especially the stage, *the documentation is not* complete.

. If upon review the unit RN, the wound nurse, or the doctor decide to change the name of a site, it *must* be written on the back of the flow sheet that the resident does not have a new wound—the site has just been renamed.

. If you fail to document that you are renaming a wound site, technically, it looks like you now have a new site without proper documentation. (E.g., the sacrum and coccyx are two different anatomical sites although in the same vicinity.)

. If you change the name of the site on the flow sheet, make sure it is changed on the treatment sheet, the orders, and the care plan as well.

. Every wound description should be individually written on the order, treatment administration record, flow sheet, and care plan.

. Completed wound flow sheets for each site should be stapled together and kept in the wound flow book until the site is completely healed so that it is easy to follow the history of a wound. Each of these sheets should be properly completed for the six aforementioned steps. On electronic medical records the history automatically remains.

. For residents with wounds, the wound care plans should not be removed from the care plan. If you complete an annual MDS and care plan assessment and the wounds still exist, staple the new care plan to the old to keep the wound history. On electronic medical records the history automatically remains.

If a resident is identified as high risk based on the pressure ulcer risk assessment, a preventative plan must be documented on the care plan even if the skin is intact.

Never write treatment to "affected site." There is no such anatomical site.

Nursing management should generate a weekly report of all wounds in-house to be distributed to doctors, rehab department and dietary department so all disciplines are aware of all wounds progress so they can implement and document their interdisciplinary approach.

Make sure the doctor mentions the wounds on the monthly history and physical.

All interventions implemented must be carried on the certified nursing assistant accountability record.

Nursing must review the wound consultant notes weekly. Make sure their sites and stages are consistent with the in-house documentation.

The MDS coordinator must be aware of all wounds.

All residents with wounds must be assessed for the following:

  a. The ability to turn and position themselves or assist when needed
  b. An air mattress
  c. Supplements (vitamin C, multivitamin, zinc, Pro-Stat, Ensure)
  d. Heel booties
  e. Elbow pads
  f. Foam wedges or pillows for positioning

All residents with wounds must have a standing order for Tylenol or other pain medication (per doctor's decision) half an hour to one hour before treatment as often as the treatment is done throughout the day.

Remind certified nursing assistants not to remove wound dressing during care and leave wound open. Nurse must be informed that dressing must be removed for showers or if soiled.

A treatment to a site should not be indefinite, especially when wound is not showing signs of improvement. Treatments need to be re-evaluated and changed every fourteen to twenty-eight days and as deemed necessary by the wound doctor or the primary doctor.

Wound rounds/meetings must be completed weekly by the interdisciplinary team of doctor, nurse, wound consultant, rehab department, and dietitian.

A weekly skin assessment should be completed on all residents in the facility and documented on the treatment administration record.

Community Acquired Wounds

1. Upon admission, all wounds must be accounted for.
2. The unit RN manager and/or the wound care RN must do a full body check on residents the next morning to ensure that no pressure ulcers were missed upon admission.
3. An individualized wound flow sheet, care plan, and treatment order must be initiated for each site.
4. Again, make sure the site, stage, size, location, place of origin, date of admission, tissue type and drainage are clearly written on each sheet.
5. Make sure to draw in wound sites on the body picture if the admission assessment has a body chart.
6. Supplements should be initiated to promote healing.
7. MDS must reflect all wounds.
8. Care plan must be completed.

Nosocomial or In-House Acquired Wounds

1. All nosocomial wounds require an accident/incident report and investigation to rule out whether or not it is avoidable or unavoidable.
2. A comprehensive nursing note should be written by an RN with particular attention to (a) residents' comorbidities (e.g., diabetes, cancer, swelling or edema etc.); (b) dietary intake; (c) recent weight lost or gained; (d) resident's behavior (refusal for perineal care or turning and positioning); (e) acute condition (e.g., diarrhea); (f) any recent decrease in mobility; (g) any devices that are contributory (e.g., oxygen tubing behind ears, tight shoes, braces, Foley pressing on labia or penis); and (h) history of healed ulcers to this site.
3. **NOTE: Initial discovery of a wound above a stage 2 is considered neglect and is reportable to the department of health! And aside from a thorough investigation, disciplinary action must ensue.**
4. A wound can *deteriorate* up to stage 3 or 4 in-house, but there must be clear documentation on the weekly flow sheets that

despite of all the interventions in place, the wound continues to deteriorate. Also mention the comorbidities.
5. Make sure the wound care consultant documentation is consistent with nursing documentation.
6. MDS must reflect all wounds.
7. Care plan must be completed.
8. The MDS coordinator must be informed of *all* nosocomial wounds to assess for a significant change.

State surveyors will look for the following:

a. Will review all required documentation to ensure completion and accuracy e.g. accident/incident report and investigation for a nosocomial ulcer, admission history, wound flow sheets, doctor's orders, treatment administration records, minimum data set (MDS) accuracy, care plan completion, certified nursing assistant accountability records and interdisciplinary progress notes.
b. During treatment observation, will monitor the resident for any signs of pain
c. Monitor to make sure the Resident's plan of care is consistently maintained on all shifts e.g. repositioning, toileting and pressure relieving devices are in place.
d. Will look at the wound and compare to the description in the documentation.
e. Check to see if the family is aware of the Resident's plan of care
f. Resident's response to interventions and treatment
g. Ensure that nurses are properly trained on wound dressing techniques with strict adherence to infection guidelines.
h. Does the resident exhibit pain during wound care.

Potential tag: F157—Physician Notified of Changes to Resident's Condition
Potential tag: F272—Comprehensive Assessment
Potential tag: F279—Comprehensive Care Plan Develop
Potential tag: F280—Care Plan Revision
Potential tag: F281—Services Provided Meet Professional Standards
Potential tag: F309—Provide Care/Services for highest Well being

Potential tag: F314—Treatment / Services to Prevent / Heal Pressure Ulcers

Potential tag: F353—Sufficient Nursing Staff on a 24 Hour Basis

Potential tag: F385—Resident Care Supervised by a Physician

Potential tag: F501—Responsibilities of the Medical Director

TRANSCRIBING DOCTOR'S ORDERS

When obtaining doctors' orders, nurses should remember "if it is not clear to you, it is most likely not clear to the other nurse" so take the time and clarify all orders!

All orders must be transcribed to the appropriate medical record and a clear precise nursing note written on what was ordered and why. Failure to appropriately transcribe all orders in the appropriate medical record can lead to delay or lack of the appropriate level of care.

Medications must be transcribed on the medication administration record.

a. Check the route, time, dosage and frequency
b. Check patient allergies and write same on the order.
c. If there is an end date or a schedule other than daily, make sure the medication administration record is boxed off appropriately.
d. For pain medications, they must be started immediately. If the ordered medication is not available doctor must be notified so readily available analgesic can be given
e. For antibiotics, they must be started within four hours of the doctor order. If the prescribed antibiotic is not readily available, get order from doctor to give another antibiotic until it arrives from the pharmacy and document same.
f. All medications must have a diagnosis written on the order and on the medication administration record!
g. Make sure the diagnosis is appropriate for the prescribed medication.
h. If an order is not clear to you, call the doctor and verify.

Treatments must be transcribed on the treatment administration record.

a. Treatments must be to an anatomical site, not "affected site."

b. If there are two treatments to the same site, there must be clear instructions on whether they can be mixed and which to apply first.

c. Treatment orders to different sites should be written separately on the orders, treatment administration records, wound flow sheets, and care plans so as they heal or treatments are changed, this can be done individually.

All diets should be transcribed on the certified nursing assistant accountability record.

All restraints should be documented on the treatment administration record and on the certified nursing assistant accountability record.

All rehab orders—e.g., start or end of therapy, devices, ambulation programs, level of care, splints, etc.—must be on the certified nursing assistants' accountability record.

Fluid restriction must be on the medication administration record and certified nursing assistant accountability record, with a breakdown sheet from the dietitian in front of them on how much fluid is provided by dietary department with meals and how much by nursing department with medications on each shift.

Extra fluid by mouth (PO), via gastrostomy tube (GT) or intravenous (IV) must be on the medication administration record.

Vent, tracheostomy, and oxygen orders must be on the treatment administration records and the certified nursing assistant accountability record.

Contact precaution or isolation must be on the treatment administration record, medication administration record, and certified nursing assistant accountability record.

Side rails must be on the treatment administration records and certified nursing assistant accountability record.

JANE GABBIDON

Alarms, floor mats, etc. (if you write orders for them) must be on certified nursing assistant accountability record.

Labs on the lab sheet and on the twenty-four-hour nursing report for follow-up until results are received and addressed by the doctor.

X-rays/diagnostic studies on the requisition forms and on the twenty-four-hour nursing report for follow-up until results are received and addressed by the doctor.

Out on pass orders must be documented on the 24 hour nursing report.

Room change orders and discharge orders must be documented on the 24 hour nursing report.

When orders are written for all the aforementioned, it is prudent for them to be carried on the twenty-four-hour nursing report to ensure all incoming nurses are aware of changes to resident's plan of care.

MDS must reflect the aforementioned.

Care plan must be completed for any order or change in resident's condition.

Family must be notified of all changes to the Resident's plan of care and this must be documented.

The following items, when accounted for on orders, must be on the treatment administration records and the certified nursing assistant accountability record:

Certified Nursing Assistant Accountability Record Should Read

a.	Oxygen	Report any SOB to nurse
b.	Vents/Tracheostomy	Report any respiratory distress to nurse
c.	Gastrostomy tubes (GT)	GT feed—keep HOB elevated 35–45 degrees

d.	Restraints	Type of Restraint; Release schedule, including mealtimes
e.	Side rails	Side rails up at HS
f.	Care items	Shampoos must follow shower days. Creams and special mouthwash must show frequency
g.	Air mattresses	Ensure mattress is inflated
h.	Devices/splints	Type, application and removal schedule
i.	Alarms	Ensure alarm is working
j.	Thickened liquids	Consistency
k.	Diagnosis of diabetes	Need to reflect that resident is diabetic
l.	Foley/Suprapubic/Urostomy	Catheter care q shift; report output to nurse
m.	Fluid restrictions	Amount of fluid resident is to receive every shift
n.	Contact precautions/Isolation	Reason for resident being on precautions
o.	Ace bandages	Application and removal schedule
p.	Hearing aids	Application and removal schedule
q.	Wander bracelets	Limb applied to and system to check it daily.

Potential tag: F514—Resident's Records must be Complete and Accurate

MEDICATION ERRORS

Most medication errors can be eliminated if nurses simply take the time to:

a. Follow the rights of medication administration: right resident, right medication, right dose, right route, right time, right reason for medication administration, no allergy to the medication and subsequent documentation.
b. Read the manufacturer's guidelines
c. Clarify orders that are confusing
d. Triple checking orders for minor but detrimental changes e.g. 2.5mg versus 25mg.
e. Signing the medication administration record immediately after giving the medication
f. Ensure proper transcription of the doctor's order.

Medication errors can be detrimental to residents. Every effort should be made to ensure that all "medication rights" are adhered to when transcribing doctors' orders or administering medications.

A facility's medication error rate must be less than 5%.

Medication errors must be accounted for on a medication error form.

The doctor must be notified of all medication errors so he or she can assess the resident for any adverse effects, and then document.

Medication error must be signed off by the Director of Nursing, the primary care doctor, and the medical director and licensed pharmacist.

If the medication error results in harm to the resident or it is a narcotic error, these are reportable to the Department of Health,

Bureau of Narcotic Enforcement and the State Licensing Board and local law enforcement (as necessary).

If a medication error is being reported, the state-required form must be completed and submitted to the Department of Health, Bureau of Narcotic Enforcement (if a narcotic), and the Attorney General's office and the Office of Professional Licensing.

Some common medication errors are:

1. Not following manufacturer's instructions e.g. shake well or don't crush'
2. Omission of doses
3. Overdosing or under-dosing
4. Medications been given without a doctor's order
5. Resident receiving wrong medications
6. Wrong dosage of medication
7. Wrong route of administration
8. Wrong medication that have similar names
9. Not administering at the right time. E.g. Synthroid should be given in early am before breakfast, never in the evening.
10. Not providing adequate fluids with medications per manufacturer's guideline
11. Medication that should be taken with food is given without
12. Not checking GT placement
13. GT flushes not done per doctor order
14. Not administering GT meds separately and flushing between each med per doctor order
15. Not ensuring eye drops make contact with the conjunctival sac
16. **Single dose vials and insulin pens not individually labelled and used individually**
17. Medications order for before or after meals given on the wrong time schedule
18. Alternating doses on different days not appropriately boxed off on the medication administration records.

NOTE: If a medication order is not clear to you, be certain it is not clear to the next nurse also so call the doctor and clarify the order!

Potential tag: F332—Free of Medication Error Rates of 5 Percent or More
Potential tag: F333—Residents are Free of Significant Medication Errors
Potential tag: F441—Infection Control

EXPIRED MEDICATIONS

Administration of expired medications is a medication error. Personnel responsible for house stock medications should ensure all medications received from vendors and delivered to nursing units are not expired.

. As part of the daily check, nurses should ensure there are no expired medications on the units or in the medication carts.

. Nurses must check all medications received from the stock room for expiration dates.

. Medications that are expiring first should be placed in the front of the storage cabinet.

. Multi-dose vials on units must have open and discard dates written on them so nurses discard in a timely manner.

. It is advisable to discard all opened vials after 28 days.

. All medications should be checked for expiration date prior to opening for patient usage.

. All emergency boxes on the nursing units or in the nursing office should be checked every shift for expired medications and should be sent to the pharmacy for replacement before any of these medications expire.

. Prior to hanging intravenous medications, nurses must always check the expiration date.

. Prior to hanging any tube feedings, the expiration date must also be checked.

. Although not a medication, facility must ensure that the AED machine (automated external defibrillator) pads are not expired.

. Saline and other dressing solutions must be checked for expiration date and must have an "open by" and "discard by" date.

. **NOTE: During survey, along with the refrigerators, medication storage is one of the first areas surveyors check looking for expired medications!**

Potential tag: F332—Free of Medication Error Rates of 5 Percent or More

Potential tag: F333—Residents are Free of Significant Medication Errors

Potential Tag: F431—drug records, label/store drugs and biologicals

PSYCHOTROPIC MEDICATION

Psychiatric medications which are also referred to as psychotropic medications are used to treat mental disorders such as depression, anxiety disorders, bipolar disorders, schizophrenia and insomnia. These medications often improve the quality of life for our residents but often have adverse side effects and can lead to dependency. There are several categories of these medications but they are collectively referred to as psychotropic medications. Categories are:

a. Antipsychotic—Mainly used to treat psychosis, schizophrenia, and bipolar e.g. Haldol, Risperdal, Zyprexia, Seroquel, Abilify
b. Antianxiety—Used for treatment of anxiety disorders e.g. Xanax, Klonopin, Valium and Ativan
c. Antidepressants—Use to manage signs/symptoms of depression e.g. Celexa, Remeron, Zoloft, Lexapro, Buspar
d. Hypnotics—Use as sleep aides-e.g. Ambien

In health care facilities, excessive psychotropic medication usage is considered chemical restraint in the absence of proper indication for usage and benefits. These medications cannot be used for the convenience of the staff.

E.g. writing that a resident was given psyche medication prn due to frequently yelling at staff is wrong. However, Resident with prolonged yelling which is preventing other residents from sleeping is okay.

Documentation must clearly reflect the effectiveness of controlling the medical symptom resident is exhibiting.

1. Make sure that with each psychiatric consult has a section on the consult report for the psychiatrist to document his attempt at gradual dose reduction (GDR).
2. Psychotropic medications *should* have the *textbook definition* for usage. (E.g., Remeron does stimulate appetite, but the primary

use is as antidepressant. Xanax does control agitation, but the primary use is as anxiolytic. And Trazodone does work for insomnia, but the primary use is as antidepressant.)

3. **NOTE**: Surveyors will cite a facility for psychotropic medications having the wrong diagnosis! E.g. Aricept and Nameda are the drugs used to treat dementia and often facilities have a lot of the other psychotropic medications documented as being used to treat dementia!

4. A full house review of all psychotropic medications should be done monthly by each unit manager. The easiest way is to have the pharmacy provide a full report of all residents on all categories of psychotropic medications or for facilities with electronic medical records, generate an internal report.

5. If the medication is been used for an off label purpose, must have clear documentation what it is been used for and why.

6. Prolonged usage of psychotropic medications requires behavior notes to show that the reason for usage still exists or to state that with the medications the resident is calm or has improved quality of life.

7. If nurses are writing that the resident is not exhibiting any behavior but remains on psychotropic medications, the psychiatrist must document on his GDR why he will not attempt to reduce the medications.

8. *Ambien usage*: If it is necessary, the starting dose should be 5mg. If you have residents on 10mg, the psychiatrist must have clear gradual dose reduction (GDR) notes.

9. NOTE: Doctor's orders for narcotics should start off with a lower dosage then subsequently increase as resident's needs change.

10. Be mindful of residents on several medications to treat the same diagnosis—e.g., Remeron, Celexa, and Trazodone to treat depression.

11. Remember, psychotropic medications affect appetite (some increase it—e.g., Remeron—and some decrease it—e.g., Seroquel and several can cause dehydration or electrolyte imbalance).

12. When residents have significant weight loss or gain, their usage of psychotropic medications should be reviewed and addressed in the documentation.
13. If a resident is on medications for dementia (i.e., Aricept and Namenda) and the resident is documented as *fully* demented, this will be viewed as unnecessary medication, so these residents need to be evaluated for possible discontinuation of the medication.
14. If a resident started exhibiting a new behavior the documentation must clearly reflect what alternate medical work-ups were done before initiating psychotropic medications.
15. The care plan must accurately reflect all behaviors displayed by resident. Nurses have a tendency to 'normalize' behaviors. E.g. A resident repeatedly picking at his nose is not a 'normal' behavior. Document it so in the event of a nose bleed this can be looked at as a possible cause
16. Doctors must remember certain medications have the potential to cause clinically adverse consequences and require routine labs for monitoring. E.g. Clozaril which is used to treat schizophrenia must have weekly blood work done.
17. Residents on psychotropic medications with decline in the ADL functions, activity intolerance and fatigue must be assessed to rule out adverse consequences of the medication.
18. **NOTE:** If there are discrepancies to psychotropic medication orders, unaddressed documented adverse reactions surveyors will review the consultant pharmacist documentation to see if this was identified and not properly addressed by the primary doctor.
19. **NOTE:** It is important for the doctor to review all psychotropic medications with each monthly assessment of the resident, especially when there are acute medical, physical or psychological changes to the resident's condition.
20. MDS must clearly reflect correct category of medication.
21. Care plan must be completed.

PRN Psychotropic Medication Usage

1. When prn (as needed) psychotropic medication usage is required, the nursing documentation must *always* state *all* other non-pharmacological interventions attempted before resorting to chemical restraint. (E.g., Resident extremely agitated. Resident was moved to a different environment; soothing music turned on. Staff attempted TLC; one-to-one attention provided. A snack was provided; however, despite of all the aforementioned, resident remains extremely agitated, so prn Ativan was given.)
2. PRN medication should not be documented as given for the benefit of staff. If the resident is combative, yes, they are a danger to staff, but they are also a danger to their self, secondary to the potential for injury. Therefore, documentation should read that resident is "a danger to self and others," with specific mention to the behaviors and the potential outcomes and, again, any non-pharmacological interventions used before medication administration.
3. Follow-up documentation is always required to include the effect/outcome of the medication.
4. Therefore, whenever a resident is given a PRN psychotropic medication, they should be documented on the twenty-four-hour nursing report and in the chart.

There are many side effects to psychotropic medications which in conjunction with our residents list of comorbidities place them at increased risk for other complications such as accident/incident, weight lost/gain and infections. Some of the more common side effects are:

a). Dizziness
b). Blurred vision
c). Increased heart rate
d). Drowsiness
e). Sensitivity to sunlight
f). Increased agitation
g). Decrease of white blood cells.

NOTE: If a resident has a sudden change in mood or behavior such as depression, sleep pattern disturbance, aggression, impaired verbal communication etc. he/she should be assessed for potential stressors such as placement in a long term care facility, feeling of loss of independence, death of a loved one, change of roommate. The resident should be assessed by a psychologist (if resident is not cognitively impaired) and/or a psychiatrist before adding or increasing psychotropic medications.

Potential tag: F154—Informed of Health Status Care and Treatment

Potential tag: F155—Right to Refuse Treatment

Potential tag: F222—Right to be Free from Chemical Restraint

Potential tag: F272—Comprehensive Assessment

Potential tag: F279—Develop Comprehensive Care Plan

Potential tag: F280—Revision of Comprehensive Care Plan

Potential tag: F310—ADLS did not Decline Unless Unavoidable

Potential tag: F319—Mental Psychological Treatment

Potential tag: F320—No Behavioral Changes Unless Unavoidable

Potential tag: F325—Maintain Nutritional Status Unless Unavoidable

Potential tag: F327—Facility Provide Sufficient Fluid to Maintain Hydration

Potential tag: F385—Resident Care Supervised by a Physician

Potential tag: F329—Drug Regimen is Free from Unnecessary Drugs

Potential tag: F501—Responsibilities of the Medical Director

ANTICOAGULANTS

Anticoagulants are blood thinners that are used to reduce formation of blood clots which can lead to heart attacks, strokes or deep vein thrombosis (clots in the deep veins of the legs impeding blood circulation). Residents on anticoagulants are at increased risk for bleeding which can be internal and not readily detected. These medications are:

Heparin
Pradaxa
Xarelto
Eliquis
Coumadin

Coumadin is the most prevalently used of these anticoagulants and like all medications have the potential for adverse effects.

a. All residents on Coumadin should have a doctor's order and a schedule for bloodwork of PT and INR a minimum of weekly.
b. Since these labs are done early in the morning, the results are usually available for early afternoon. Therefore, there should be an assigned nurse who follows up to ensure all results are received and discussed with the doctor in a timely manner. (This applies to *all* labs.)
c. If a new dose of Coumadin is ordered, it is advisable for the doctor to discontinue the previous dose, not put it on hold. **Note:** The doctor should not put any medication on hold indefinitely.
d. When orders are written for alternating doses of Coumadin, they must be very clear to avoid medication errors.
e. Write alternating doses as two separate orders with the days to be given as part of the order. Make sure the medication administration record is properly boxed off.

f. Must have a system for standard weekly labs that is accessible and clear for all nurses to follow when the regular nurse is off duty.

g. Any Coumadin order changes and scheduled repeat labs should be carried on the twenty-four-hour nursing report to ensure follow-through.

h. A nursing note should *always* be written regarding *all* lab results received, even if they are normal.

i. If the doctor makes recommendations regarding the lab results, it is good advice to write these recommendations on the lab and then write an order.

j. If there are no recommendations from the doctor, write this on the lab result and in the nursing notes also.

k. Residents on Coumadin with any form of bleeding should be addressed with the doctor promptly (e.g., bleeding gums when brushing teeth).

l. Vitamin K is the drug given when Coumadin levels are too high (as per doctor's parameters). It must be readily available in the emergency drug box on nursing units.

NOTE: Green leafy vegetables contain vitamin K and too much vitamin K lowers the effect of Coumadin.

Because of the increased risk of bleeding, residents on anticoagulants should be closely monitored for:

> Bleeding gums especially when brushing teeth
> Nose bleeds
> Coffee ground vomiting
> Bleeding on the brain in the event of head injury (note by a sudden or gradual change in mental status baseline)
> Excessive bleeding from injection sites
> Dark colored urine
> Post-menopausal vaginal bleeding
> Dark tarry stools

It is advisable to have a separate Coumadin medication administration record and the weekly PT/INR results written in on the back.

		1	2	3	4	5	6
Date	Coumadin _____mg At bedtime						
Date	Coumadin _____mg At bedtime						
Date	Coumadin _____mg At bedtime						

Care plan must be completed.

MDS should reflect appropriate diagnosis

NOTE: In the event of harm or death to a resident as a result of anticoagulant usage, the State will request the facility's protocol which must clear reflect how often PT and INR are done, system for timely notifying the doctor of lab results, system for holding the medication, system for follow-up labs, system for monitoring for adverse reactions such as bleeding and timeliness of the response!

Potential tag: F279—Develop Comprehensive Care Plan

Potential tag: F505—Promptly Notify Physician of Lab Results

HANDLING OF CONTROLLED SUBSTANCES

Controlled medications which the healthcare industry refers to as narcotics, are tightly regulated by the government because of the potential for abuse. The Drug Enforcement Administration (DEA) is the federal regulator of controlled medications. In New York State, the Bureau of Narcotic Enforcement (BNE) is the regulatory body responsible for combating any illegal diversion of prescription controlled medications.

NOTE: Nurses should be mindful that narcotic errors are also reportable to the Licensing Board! Narcotic diversion affects every nurse that is responsible for handling them!

In an effort to combat narcotic diversion, facilities must have an efficient system for tracking narcotics from the time they enter the facility until they are administered or destroyed.

NOTE: When doing narcotics count, because of the possibility of narcotic diversion, check the back of the blister pack to make sure no pills are taped in and all pills look the same!

NOTE: Narcotics must be counted TOGETHER by two nurses at all times, even if it is for a simple exchange of keys during a break or a change of unit!!

NOTE: Nurses have to be mindful that once they take the keys, they are accountable and must take responsibility for *all* manifested narcotic violations and errors!!

NOTE: Narcotic reconciliation book should have a clear account of all residents on controlled substances, and books must be signed every shift by oncoming and off-going nurse TOGETHER!!!

Together means together! Both nurses should look at the count on the record together; count the pills together; check the blister packs together and thereafter sign the record to give authenticity to the counting!

Narcotics must always be stored at a minimum behind double-locked doors.

Narcotics in the medication cart must be in a locked bin in the locked cart.

NOTE: The record of emergency supply of narcotics must be counted every shift by the oncoming and off-going RN supervisors together and like all other narcotics, this must be properly secured with clear documentation of usage, waste and destruction

If narcotics require refrigeration, the facility must have a locked box in the medication fridge that is chained into the fridge.

The shelves in the narcotic refrigerator must be bolted into the refrigerator also.

When residents are transferred to a hospital or discharged, nurses should promptly return the unused narcotics to the director of nursing/designee to promote accountability and prevent violations.

Narcotic waste must be witnessed and signed for by the medication nurse and an RN supervisor.

Narcotic medication error form must be signed by the doctor, the director of nursing, the administrator, licensed pharmacist and the medical director.

Narcotic medication errors are reportable to the Department of Health, Bureau of Narcotic and Licensing Board and possible local law enforcement.

Facility must ensure prescription pads are stored in a secure location and must have a system in place for logging prescriptions written by the doctor and safeguarding until delivered to the pharmacy personnel.

The following are possible narcotic violations that could generate citations from the State:

a. Nurses not counting narcotics together
b. Unreported wrong counts
c. Unreported missing narcotics
d. Un-witnessed destruction of narcotics
e. Failure to count at the start or end of a shift
f. Failure to remove unused narcotics from the narcotic box after discharge or discontinuation of medication
g. Fraudulent reconciliation

Potential tag: F431: Proper drug Records, Labelling and Storage of Drugs and Biologicals

USAGE AND STORAGE OF INSULIN

Diabetes is a condition that causes increase in the blood sugar because of the body's inability to produce insulin in sufficient quantities. There are two types of diabetes: a). Type 1 diabetes is when the pancreas does not produce any insulin. B) Type 2 diabetes is when the body produces insulin but does not use it properly.

Type 1 diabetics require insulin injections. Type 2 diabetics often require medications referred to as oral hypoglycemic medications. Residents on these medications require ongoing monitoring.

1. All residents on insulin or oral hypoglycemic medications should have a schedule for blood glucose monitoring.
2. The doctor should have a schedule for periodic blood draw-HgA1C.
3. Diabetic residents who have finger-stick orders without insulin or oral hypoglycemic medications need to have parameters as to when to notify doctor—e.g., if blood sugar is below 70mg/dl or above 120mg/dl, notify doctor.
4. For residents who receive insulin on a sliding scale, it is advisable for the facility to have a standard sliding scale per policy to minimize medication errors such as wrong dosage administration or errors in transcription.
5. Medication administration record should reflect the site injection was given and the amount of insulin given (if on a sliding scale).
6. Injection sites should be rotated.
7. When there are multiple residents on insulin, each must have his or her own vial individually bagged and staff must be trained to draw insulin from individual bottles for each resident and administer it based on resident' specific order.
8. Insulin vials *must* be dated once opened. The opening date and the date it should be discarded must be clearly marked on the vials.

9. Advisable to discard open vials within 28 days.
10. It is advisable to have a check-off form for RN supervisors to check insulin daily for dates and expiration as a backup to the nurses on the units.
11. Insulin must be stored in a locked medication refrigerator at a temperature of 36 to 46 degrees.
12. Insulin must be given at room temperature so it must be removed from the refrigerator and allowed to warm up prior to administration.
13. Certified nursing assistant accountability record must reflect if a resident is diabetic.
14. Dietary must ensure that there are snacks available for diabetics at nights.
15. Recreation department, dietary and in-house café staff must be aware of all diabetic residents.
16. It is advisable that diabetic residents can be easily identified by wearing color ID bands specific to diabetic residents in your building or other facility preferred identifier.

MDS must reflect diabetic status.

Care plan must be completed.

NOTE: Be aware that residents with diabetes are at risk for foot ulcers hence it is advisable to put in place proper foot wear, regular podiatry visits and other appropriate interventions.

NOTE: For residents receiving insulin injections or ANY injections daily, surveyors will check:

a. Administration technique such as cleansing of site, proper route, infection control such as hand washing, gloving etc.
b. Are injection sites rotated and is this documented (MUST be a part of the instructions written on the medication administration record).
c. Proper disposal of syringes and needles. (Ensure sharp containers are in place and not fill above the required line!).
d. Resident privacy maintained when giving injections

e. Assess resident for pain, swelling, redness from previous injections.

Potential tag: F272—Comprehensive Assessment

Potential tag: F279—Develop Comprehensive Care Plan

Potential tag: F280—Revision of Comprehensive Care Plan

Potential tag: F328—Treatment/Care for Special Care Needs

Potential tag: F441—infection Control

UNIT REFRIGERATORS

Too often there is confusion as to whether nursing or maintenance is responsible for the unit refrigerators. Nurses use these refrigerators to store medications and food and they are locked in the medication room. Therefore, they are the responsibility of the nursing department. Also during survey, the nurses are the ones who are questioned about them so nursing should monitor them.

1. Nursing units should have two refrigerators. One fridge is for medications only, and one is for food items.
2. Medications and food items should never be mixed.
3. All food items in the pantry fridge must have a name and date.
4. All multi-dose vials in the medication fridge must have a label for open and discard dates.
5. If there are narcotics that require refrigeration, the facility must have a locked box that is chained or properly secured in the locked medication refrigerator in the locked medication room. The narcotic refrigerator shelves must also be bolted in the fridge.
6. Refrigerator temperature must be monitored and recorded on a log daily and must reflect a range of 36 to 46 degrees.
7. Must have a system in place for checking the temperature in both refrigerators.
8. There must be a defrosting and cleaning schedule in place for all refrigerators.
9. Upon entering the facility for survey, the refrigerator and the accompanying logs are one of the first areas surveyors look at.

The most common citations in this area:

a. staff leaving personal undated food items in the refrigerators
b. Staff not ensuring fridge temperature is in the correct range
c. Staff not properly maintaining the refrigerator logs
d. Narcotic storage without the shelves been bolted.

Potential tag: F431—Drug records, Label/Store Drugs & Biologicals

ACCIDENTS AND INCIDENTS

An accident is an unexpected or unintended event, especially one resulting in human injury or death. An incident is an unplanned event that did not result in injury.

An accident/incident report is an important tool used to narrate the details of what, where, whom, when and how of an occurrence. It is important to report and investigate all accidents/incidents because minor incidents can worsen over time and lead to injury.

All accident/incident reports should be followed up with an investigation to rule out whether <u>abuse, neglect</u> or <u>mistreatment</u> occurred. (Accident and incident reports are completed for instances involving employees, but for this discussion, the focus is on accident/incident for a resident).

A fall risk assessment must be completed on all residents on

1. Admission
2. With any accident/incident
3. Quarterly
4. With any significant change.

Accidents/incidents require an assessment which by scope of practice can only be done by an RN. Therefore,

a. The nurse on the unit must write a statement and a note in the resident's progress notes.
b. The RN supervisor on duty must assess the resident and also write a statement and a note in the resident's progress notes.
c. It is advisable that the accident/incident form be completed by the RN supervisor.

The doctor and family must be notified at the time of accident/incident and this must be clearly documented, with preferably the name of the family member spoken with identified in the notes.

If it is documented that the nurse was unable to reach the family at the time of an incident, this information must be documented on the 24 hour nursing report for follow-up until it is documented that the family was contacted. This should be clearly documented in the nursing notes.

Nurses should be encouraged that when there is an accident/incident, they should look at the interventions in place, assess the situation thoroughly, before writing the report. (E.g., Writing "On rounds, I saw the resident lying on the floor" when in fact the resident has a bed alarm, which you heard while making rounds and responded to. Or "Resident noted on floor" when in fact resident has floor mats and was lying on same.)

Nurses should be precise in their documentation (e.g., "resident found on floor—sitting, kneeling, lying on which side?).

Nurses should always state the position of the head in relation to the floor to rule out whether or not resident hit his/her head during the fall. When in doubt about head injury promptly initiate neuro checks!

Nurses should review all statements and documentation regarding the accident/incident and ensure consistency before submission to the director of nursing/designee. (e.g., a bruise, laceration, abrasion, skin tear are all different).

Statements should be obtained from the nurse on the unit, the RN supervisor, the certified nursing assistant assigned to the resident and any staff member who witnessed or reported the incident.

The RN should update the care plan on the shift the accident/incident occurs with new interventions and attach a copy of that care plan with the submitted accident/incident report.

The fall risk assessment and the pain assessment should be completed also and a copy attached to the accident/incident report.

New interventions must be updated on the certified nursing assistant accountability record also and dated for the time of the incident.

Encourage nurses not to put unrealistic goals (e.g., resident will be on 1:1—unless there is a true 1:1; resident will be kept close to nursing station at all times—what about at nights?)

Nurses must write a note regarding *the* accident/incident in the doctor's communication book so he or she is aware the next morning to assess the resident and write a progress note.

NOTE: Every resident with an accident/incident must be access by the doctor no later than 48 hours and a note written. If resident was transferred to the hospital or discharged, MD must write that he/she was unable to assess resident as resident was hospitalized or discharge.

NOTE: If a resident experienced an accident/incident as a result of being restrained, particular attention must be paid to the risks versus benefits of ongoing restraint usage. E.g. a resident with full side rails becomes entrapped by the rails. Probably it is best to remove rails and give resident a low positioned bed with floor mats and an alarm.

NOTE: The primary reason for doing an accident/incident report and investigation is to rule out whether abuse, neglect, or mistreatment occurred and to determine if it is reportable to the Department of Health. Therefore the facility's investigation form must address:

1. Where there is abuse, neglect or mistreatment
2. Whether or not an accident/incident was reported to the Department of Health.

To ensure that all accidents/incidents are thoroughly investigated and concluded, it is advisable that the Director of Nursing/assistant director of nursing/risk manager review and conclude all accidents/incidents.

Accidents/incidents requires an interdisciplinary approach. Therefore, it is advisable to have a form that can be signed by all the necessary disciplines. It is advisable to have the following disciplines involved: (a) nursing service, (b) rehab department, (c) primary care doctor, (d) medical director, (e) social services and (f) administrator.

When concluding an accident/incident investigation, it is advisable that you compare the accident/incident report, all statements, the note documented in the medical records, and what interventions are already in place on the certified nursing assistant accountability record and the care plan.

If the statements are not consistent with the incident, staff can write a clarification statement that must be attached to their original statement.

If the interviewer receives a verbal clarification via telephone from a staff member, he or she can write that verbal clarification and indicate on it that "it is a verbal clarification from the staff member," in the presence of a witness. Interviewer should read back the individual's statement and indicate on it that it was read back.

Reporting of accidents/incidents to the Department of Health must be by the state guidelines in a timely manner. Therefore stress on nurses the importance of completing accident/incident report in a timely manner.

All accident/incidents must have interventions implemented. Some residents may have excessive accidents/incidents and it may seem there are no other interventions to implement. In some instances, a goal to prevent injury may be the only feasible option with similar interventions.

All staff should be aware that doors that are self-closing, leading to hazardous areas and to corridors, must be kept closed at all times, including shower rooms and pantries. Do not use door jars to keep them open. (Although this falls under fire and safety, it creates the potential for an accident/incident)

When a resident is injured while at an outside appointment, upon return resident must be fully assessed, family and doctor notified, accident/incident report completed and statements obtained from all outsiders including the ambulette crew.

Accident/incident prevention is a mandatory in-service and all staff should be aware of potential hazards in the environment.

NOTE: Whenever there is an accident/incident, a systematic review needs to be done to rule out the possibility of other residents been affected. E.g. a resident sustained a skin tear from the arm rest of the w/c. The arm rests of all w/c should be checked for sharp edges.

Care plan must be completed.

MDS must reflect falls.

To clearly rule out whether any situation constitutes abuse, neglect, or mistreatment, it is highly recommended that an accident/incident be done for all the preceding instances. Although it may seem excessive, it is actually a good tool to know what is going on in a facility.

1. Falls (witnessed or unwitnessed)
2. Lowered to the floor by staff
3. Bruises
4. Abrasions
5. Lacerations
6. Skin tears
7. Areas of discoloration
8. Areas of swelling
9. Fractures
10. Resident-to-resident verbal altercation
11. Resident-to-resident physical altercation
12. Smoking in unauthorized areas
13. Elopement
14. Dislodged Foleys
15. Dislodged tracheostomy
16. Dislodged GT
17. Dislodged IV tubing (especially central and PICC lines)
18. Sexual encounters or exposure

19. Choking incidents
20. Burns
21. Medication error
22. Injury of unknown origin
23. Suicide attempted or death related to suicide/restraints/equipment
24. Staff-to-resident abuse
25. Family/visitor-to-resident abuse
26. Misappropriation of resident property
27. Ingestion of non-food items (pica)

NOTE: Residents expressing suicidal ideation must be monitored on every fifteen minutes rounds. If the resident has an expressed or witnessed plan for committing the act, resident must be maintained on 1:1 monitoring until transfer to hospital.

Potential tag: F221—Right to Free from Physical Restraints

Potential tag: F223—Right to be Free from Abuse

Potential tag: F272—Comprehensive Assessment

Potential tag: F279—Comprehensive Care Plan

Potential tag: F280—Comprehensive Care Plan Revision

Potential tag: F281—Services Provided Meet Professional Standards

Potential tag: F323—Free of Accident Hazards/Supervision/Devices

Potential tag: F353—Sufficient Nursing Staff 24 Hours a Day

Potential tag: F520—Quality Assessment & Assurance (accident prevention)

ELOPEMENT

There are various definitions of elopement. In law, elopement is an act of secretly leaving home to marry without parental consent. In healthcare, elopement is the departure of a patient from a psychiatric unit or hospital without permission. In correction facilities, elopement is slang for the escape of an inmate. In a nursing home, elopement is the departure of a resident without permission or without escort from the facility.

Elopement is considered a serious violation and it can rise to the level of immediate jeopardy. One of the cause of elopement in a nursing home is wandering.

Wandering Residents:

Every administrator and director of nursing is terrified of the dreadful call about an elopement!

Wandering places cognitively impaired residents at risk for injury. Wandering is often a purposeful behavior driven by the desire to fulfill some spoken or unspoken need or the desire to fulfill a psychological and or a physical need. E.g. to get home before dark, to pick up children at the bus stop, the urge to urinate, looking for a family member.

In an attempt to prevent elopement, the facility must clearly identify all wanderers and have a reliable system for notifying all staff of high risk residents. A wandering/elopement assessment should be done:

    a. On admission
    b. Quarterly
    c. With any significant changes in physical or mental condition.

NOTE: If a confused resident wanders into the basement or any other unsupervised area in the building or leaves the building without any direct supervision, this is considered an elopement.

NOTE: If a staff member is with a resident who wanderers into an unsafe area or even out of the building, this is not considered an elopement, as resident was directly supervised at all times.

For wanderers, the following is advisable:

a. Have a colored collage of all wanderers on every unit, in each department, and at the main desk so all staff on all units and in all departments are aware of these residents.

b. Update the collage when there are changes and redistribute as needed.

c. The form that the certified nursing assistants sign for hourly rounds should have the collage of all wanderers in the facility on top or on the back so all certified nursing assistants on all units are aware of all wanderers.

d. A copy of the collage should be in all medication administration records, all treatment records and all certified nursing assistant records and updated as needed.

e. Must have a system in place to ensure all wander bracelets are in place. They must be checked for placement and for functionality every day. The checks must also be documented!

f. If a resident who is deemed a wanderer is transferred to the Emergency Room, this should be written on the transfer form.

g. Wanders must be escorted to all outside appointments and the accompanying staff member must be aware of the wandering status.

h. If a wanderer is going out on pass with family, they should also be aware.

i. On electronic medical records, it is important to update the main screen of wanderers so that anyone logging on is aware that resident is a high risk for elopement

j. Have a system in place to check wander bracelet placement every shift and for functionality daily.

k. Resident must be clearly identified as a wanderer on the certified nursing assistant accountability record, if a wander bracelet is in place and which extremity
l. Elopement is a mandatory in-service for all staff and it is advisable for the facility to do a missing resident drill at a minimum yearly.
m. MDS must clearly reflect behavior.
n. Care plan must be completed.

NOTE: Restraining a wandering resident just to prevent wandering can be constituted as abuse. E.g. a resident who constantly wanders into other residents rooms is placed in a chair that prevents rising.

Potential tag: F221—Right to Free from Physical Restraints

Potential tag: F223—Right to be Free from Abuse

Potential tag: F272—Comprehensive Assessment

Potential tag: F279—Comprehensive Care Plan

Potential tag: F280—Comprehensive Care Plan Revision

Potential tag: F281—Services Provided Meet Professional Standards

Potential tag: F323—Free of Accident Hazards/Supervision/Devices

Potential tag: F353—Sufficient Nursing Staff 24 Hours a Day

Potential tag: F520—Quality Assessment & Assurance (accident prevention)

ABUSE, NEGLECT OR MISTREATMENT

Most cases reported to the Department of Health involve instances of abuse, neglect or mistreatment or violation of resident's rights!

Abuse can be emotional, physical, verbal or sexual. Neglect is failure to provide food, health care, medications, turning and positioning, toileting or other necessary services to vulnerable residents. Mistreatment is intentional actions of a caregiver that causes harm or the risk for harm to a resident.

The purpose for doing accidents/incidents reports and investigations is to rule out abuse, neglect or mistreatment. Therefore, it is advisable to refer to the previously mentioned list and complete an accident/incident report for all of the aforementioned areas.

Facility must have policies and procedures incorporating the seven components of abuse prevention: SPPIRIT—screen, prevent, protect, identify, report, investigate, train.

Abuse is a mandatory ongoing in-service and all staff should be aware of the various types of abuse which are verbal, physical, sexual, mental, corporal punishment and involuntary seclusion.

NOTE: As per The Centers for Medicare/Medicaid, properly trained staff should be able to respond appropriately to resident behavior. CMS does not consider striking a combative resident an appropriate response in ANY situation. Retaliation by staff is abuse!

Retaliation by using derogatory language, rough handling, ignoring resident while giving care, telling residents who need to be toileted to urinate or defecate on themselves is abuse!

Verbal abuse can be written as a grievance but must also be fully investigated.

NOTE: When there is suspected or reported abuse, the facility must act promptly to protect all residents by stopping all contact between the accuser and the accused until a full investigation is concluded.

NOTE: As part of any investigation involving abuse, the State will be reviewing the accused employee records; hence the importance of facilities ensuring that a criminal background check is done or license checks on required individuals and results received, reviewed and are present in the employee's records.

Cases of abuse should be reported to the Department of Health within 5 days of discovery.

Potential tag: F223—Right to be Free from Abuse

Potential tag: F224—Staff Treatment of Residents

Potential tag: F225—Not Employ Persons Guilty of Abuse

Potential tag: F226—Development of Abuse, Neglect etc. Policies

ELDER JUSTICE ACT

The Elder Justice Act is a Federal law to protect elderly from abuse, neglect or mistreatment. This requires reporting of any reasonable suspicion of a crime committed against a resident. This must be reported to the local law enforcement agencies and, subsequently, to the Department of Health.

In instances of staff to resident, visitor-to-resident or resident to resident physical contact, it is imperative that aside from the usual investigation and reporting to the Department of Health, local law enforcement must be notified. This should be documented in the medical records.

1. All physical altercations between residents should be reported to the Department of Health and reported to the local precinct.
2. It is the responsibility of the facility to protect its residents. Therefore even if an alert and oriented x3 resident who is being abuse by family does not want any actions taken, it is advisable for the facility to intervene by reporting the occurrence.
3. Residents returning from out on pass with families/friends with any suspicious bruises should also be thoroughly assessed and an accident/incident report and investigation must be completed to rule out abuse.
4. If a resident is been discharged to a family member per their request and there is suspicion or concern regarding abuse, it is advisable to enlist the help of the Adult Protective Agency.

NOTE: Whenever local law enforcement are called to a facility, it is important to record the names and badge numbers of the responding officers in the resident's medical records for future reference.

NOTE: Reported Allegations of unwitnessed physical abuse must be treated in the same manner due to the vulnerability of the resident!

Potential tag: F223—Free from Abuse

Potential tag: F224—Prohibit Mistreatment

Potential tag: F225—Investigate/Report Allegations/Individuals

Potential tag: F226—Development of Abuse, Neglect etc. Policies

CRIMINAL HISTORY RECORD CHECK (CHRC)

Criminal history check is often done by a clerical person but when there are issues, the director of nursing is the one who takes responsibility. Therefore, nursing management should review all paperwork to ensure compliance!

In an effort to combat abuse, neglect or mistreatment of the elderly, the Federal Government prohibits elder care facilities from hiring employees who have been found guilty of crimes against a resident. Background check is important and the system varies by state. In New York State:

. Facility must have someone who is given authority from the state agency to submit requests and view results, usually human resource, nursing management or the administrator.

. This facility representative must complete form CHRC 101 and submit it.

. If the facility designated representative has been removed, the facility must complete form CHRC 106 and submit to the state agency.

. *Who is subject to CHRC?*

All non-licensed employees providing direct care to residents/clients with any contact with residents:

    a. Certified nursing assistants (must also be screened through the nurse aide registry)
    b. Home health-care attendants
    c. Dietary aids
    d. Hairdressers and barbers
    e. Housekeepers
    f. Maintenance workers

. *Who is not subject to CHRC*: All employees licensed under NYS's education law:

a. Nursing home administrators
b. Doctors, Nurse Practitioner, Physician Assistant
c. Nurses
d. Social workers
e. Dietitians
f. Volunteers
g. Respiratory therapists

. As part of the process, the employees that are subject to CHRC must be fingerprinted.

. They must also sign a consent form-CHRC 102.

. Any newly hired employee who is subject to CHRC must be under daily documented supervision until the final results for employment determination are received from CHRC agency.

. The supervision must be performed by another employee on the same unit as the newly hired employee but need *not* be employed in the same department.

. If the new employee leaves or is terminated based on the results of CHRC, a termination form-CHRC 105 must be filed with the agency in charge of the registry and a copy is placed in the employee's record.

. CHRC agency will generally email the results to the facility's designated representative and they mail a copy of negative results to the employee also.

. CHRC results generally clear within a few days.

. If the newly hired employee has a criminal background, the results will be sent to CHRC legal for determination.

. A negative determination instructs provider to *immediately* remove from direct care.

. The results are generally e-mailed to the facility's designated representative.

. The CHRC results must remain confidential and must be retained for the facility *six years* after the person ceases to be employed by the facility.

NOTE: Surveyors generally check the files of several employees hired within the past 3-6months to ensure the facility is properly screening all new employees prior to hire.

NOTE: For licensed professionals, it is advisable to check with the Office of Professional License to ensure there are no cases of abuse, neglect or narcotic diversion etc. pending against them.

NOTE: For nurses, it is advisable to check to see if they were ever a certified nursing assistant and there were any outstanding issues of resident abuse, neglect or mistreatment.

Potential tag: F225—Not Employ Persons Guilty of Abuse

Potential tag: F495—Nurse Aid Registry Verification

Potential tag: F499—Facility Employ Qualified Professional Staff

NURSING STAFFING

Inadequate staffing not only affects staff morale, it also significantly impacts on resident care!

In the continued effort to prevent resident neglect, facilities are responsible for employing an adequate amount of staff to ensure residents daily care needs are met in accordance with their individualized plan of care.

All nurse staffing numbers for all three shifts must be posted daily in a highly visible area. The count must accurately reflect hours worked.

1. The number of RN on duty, including management RNs
2. The number of LPN on duty
3. The number of CNAs on duty, including those assigned to rehab or on escort

The facility's name and the date must be clearly visible.

Surveyors gauge a facility's staffing needs on staff and resident census ratio and:

a. Staff response to call bells
b. Are residents toileted, turned and re-positioned or ambulated in a timely manner?
c. Are residents supervised on frequent rounds?
d. Is resident receiving care according to the plan of care on every shift? e.g. two persons at all times for turning and positioning and bathing
e. Is there a licensed nurse supervising care on each shift?
f. Resident/Family complaints
g. Trends in the facility which may indicate decrease quality of care, e.g. increased accidents/incidents, nosocomial pressure ulcers

h. Increased number of residents with issues such as weight lost, decreased in activities of daily living performance
i. Sudden changes to a resident's baseline mental and physical status are properly identified and managed

NOTE: This information must be maintained and readily available for at least two years.

Potential tag: F353—Sufficient 24 Hour Nursing Staff per Care Plan Needs

Potential tag: F354—Use of Charge Nurse & Registered Nurse

Potential tag: F355—Licensed Nurses 24hr/day.

Potential tag: F356—posting nurse staffing information

IN-SERVICE TRAINING

There are required mandatory in-services for all staff but ongoing staff training on all other aspects of resident care is extremely important.

1. Facility must have system in place for ensuring ongoing education of all staff.
2. Must have a clear system of easily identifying if a particular employee received a particular in-service without having to scroll through ten pages of signatures.
3. *All* staff from all departments must be in-serviced yearly on the mandatory required in-services, which are the following:

   a. Accidents and incidents
   b. Elopement
   c. Needs of the elderly / dealing with the aggressive resident
   d. Infection control
   e. Hot and cold weather precautions
   f. Abuse
   g. Fire and safety
   h. HIPAA (Health Insurance Portability and Accountability Act--maintaining resident's privacy)

4. <u>All nursing staff should have a minimum of twelve hours of in-service trainings per calendar year</u>, including all mandatory trainings and all other pertinent areas with potential for deficient practice.
5. Daily pertinent issues that arise should be used as teaching/in-service opportunities. E.g. resident complaint of room being too cold, all staff should be in-serviced on the importance of checking thermometers when in Residents rooms. Nurse made a medication error, all nurses should be in-serviced on all components of avoiding medication errors from obtaining an order, to transcription, to accountability for medications to administration to resident.

6. Equipment usage such as Hoyer lifts, scales, and rehab devices, such as splints should be ongoing in-services for certified nursing assistants and not just once a year based on competency evaluations.

Potential tag: F497—Regular In-service Education

COMPETENCY TESTING

Return demonstration is the best way of knowing if someone grasps a skill that was taught to them!

NOTE: Facility MUST have a form in place to provide yearly competency testing for *all* certified nursing assistants. This is a regulatory requirement!

NOTE: It is also a regulatory requirement for facilities to also do a yearly evaluation on all nurses!

This form must address all aspects of their daily assignment to show they are still proficient in these areas.

For example, in the event of an injury involving the Hoyer, this is the facility's proof that a certified nursing assistant was monitored throughout the year to show they are still fully aware how to utilize all equipment safely and appropriately.

Potential tag: F495—Nurse Aid Competency

Potential tag: F497—Regular In-service Education

Potential tag: F498—Nurse Aide Demonstrates Competency/Care Needs

PHYSICAL RESTRAINTS

As per the New York State Operation Manual, the resident has the right to be free from any physical or chemical restraints imposed for purposes of discipline and convenience and not required to treat the resident's medical symptoms.

E.g. writing that a seat belt was applied because staff is constantly redirecting resident to sit down is wrong but writing that resident constantly stands and is at risk for fall with severe injury so seat belt was applied is appropriate.

Physical restraints, like chemical restraints, cannot be used for the benefit of the staff. Restraint should only be used if the resident is exhibiting behavior that puts him/her at risk for injury to self or others!

Physical restraint is defined as any device, material or equipment attached to or adjacent to the resident's body that the individual cannot remove easily and restricts freedom of movement or normal access to one's body.

All restraints that have been initiated must have the following components:

a. Interdisciplinary team (IDT) discussion, consensus and documentation on the need for the restraint.
b. Interdisciplinary team completion of the restraint device assessment form.
c. Doctor's order for type of restraint with release schedule of every two hours for fifteen minutes, at meal times and during care.
d. Signed informed consent from resident and/or family/legal representative (form must be kept in the chart).
e. Care plan, which must be signed by interdisciplinary team.
f. Clear, precise progress note as to what other interventions were in place prior to initiating the restraint.
g. Rehab department evaluation of resident and recommendation of appropriate restraint device.

All restraints and release schedule at every two hours for 15 minutes, at mealtimes and during care and should be on the treatment administration record so nurses are aware.

All restraints and release schedule should be on the order, care plan and certified nursing assistants accountability record.

For self-releasing restraints, these must be assessed frequently to ensure resident can self-release.

Restraints assessment (including self-releasing ones) must be done every *three* months at a minimum and must be clearly documented on the care plan and the progress notes that sometime during that three-month period you attempted to release/reduce the restraint and why it was not effective (e.g., "For two days we attempted to remove the seatbelt and maintained resident on close supervision. Resident was observed to be repeatedly restless and at increased risk for falls/injury).

NOTE: Due to the restrictive nature of restraints and constant changes in resident health dynamics, it is advisable for the interdisciplinary team to re-assess restraint use monthly rather than quarterly as per facility policy and every attempt made to reduce usage.

If restraint usage is necessary, it is advisable to start off with the least-restrictive restraint; e.g. before applying a seatbelt or tabletop, try a pummel cushion.

The following all meet the criteria for restraints:

a. Abdominal binders (only remove for care)
b. Mittens
c. Seatbelts (front or back closure)
d. Lapboards, tabletops or bars
e. Lap buddies
f. Wrist restraints
g. Pummel cushions
h. Merry Walker (if resident is unaware how to get out of it)
i. Certain clothing e.g. a jumpsuit

j. A chair that prevents rising for an ambulatory resident
k. Side rails (full and half-rails if resident is unable to use for turning and positioning)
l. Bed or chair against a wall to prevent resident from getting out. (Note: There are times bed may be against wall to increase the living space in the room but this must be care planned for)

Make sure ALL accounts for a restraint read the same e.g. MD order cannot say side rails are used for turning and positioning and all other accounts say unaware of bed boundary.

It is advisable for the facility to designate a restraint champion who is responsible for scheduling restraint review meetings monthly or quarterly. This could be the rehab director, assistant director of nursing or quality assurance coordinator.

MDS must reflect the restraint.

Care plan must be completed.

Potential tag: F157—Family Notification

Potential tag: F221—Right to be Free from Physical Restraints

Potential tag: F272—Comprehensive Assessment

Potential tag: F279—Develop Comprehensive Care Plan

Potential tag: F280—Revision of Comprehensive Care Plan

Potential tag: F310—ADLS did not Decline Unless Unavoidable

Potential tag: F320—No Behavioral Changes Unless Unavoidable

Potential tag: F385—Resident Care Supervised by a Physician

Potential tag: F501—Responsibilities of the Medical Director

REFUSAL OF CARE BY THE RESIDENT

A resident has the right to refuse treatment. When a resident refuses care, the following must be considered:

1. The health-care proxy has the right to make all decisions when the resident refuses, if the resident is confused.
2. If there is no health-care proxy / power of attorney, the facility must make a decision on treatment if the resident is confused. As per the New York State Operation Manual, "the resident's refusal of treatment does not absolve the facility from providing care that allows the resident to attain or maintain his/her highest level of well-being."
3. When an alert resident refuses treatment (e.g., chemotherapy, rehab, showers, daily grooming, etc.), every attempt must be made to educate and encourage the resident. If the alert resident continues to refuse, this must be care-planned for by the interdisciplinary team with ongoing documentation by the team to indicate the issue was readdressed with the resident.
4. When a resident refuses medication the doctor must be notified and this must be documented.
5. If a resident is constantly refusing a medication that they need, it is <u>not</u> advisable for the doctor to discontinue it. E.g. a very unstable diabetic resident is refusing insulin.
6. Residents who are constantly refusing care must be seen by psychiatry department and/or psychology department to asses for underlying reasons for refusal.
7. If ongoing refusal is affecting a resident's health, quality of life, or that of other residents, hospitalization may be necessary.
8. A resident cannot be discharged from a facility because they refuse treatment. E.g. an alert resident has significant weight loss but refuses a feeding tube. Ongoing teaching and family involvement should be provided and resident may be sent to hospital with the hope that the hospital doctor involvement may be beneficial.

E.g. an alert resident refusing to have his or her liquids thickened secondary to dysphasia. The facility should provide the resident with thickened liquids. However, the resident and/or the family have the right to purchase and consume thin liquids if resident desires.)

9. Care planning is crucial.
10. MDS must reflect behavior

Potential tag: F156—Rights to Refuse Treatment, Experimental Research or to Formulate Advance Directives

Potential tag: F242—Self Determination—Resident Make Choices.

ADVANCE DIRECTIVES

Residents/family/legal representative have the right to refuse to implement advance directives, even in instances when death is eminent.

On admission to a facility, social services department is responsible for resident/family/legal representative teaching on advance directives and ensuring that all required signed documents are readily available in the resident's medical records in the event of an emergency.

Advance directives are written instructions one puts in place relating to his or her care in the event the individual becomes incapacitated to make decisions. These are:

1. Health Care Proxy: Is someone appointed by an individual to speak on their behalf if they are unable to make their own healthcare decisions.
2. Living Will—Allows an individual to state their wishes about medical care in the even they develop an irreversible condition that prevents them from making their own medical decisions.
3. Surrogate—The person who has the legal authority to consent to a DNR order for an individual who lacks the capacity. E.g. Health care proxy; legal guardian; parent, spouse; son or daughter; brother or sister; close friend, physicians at the facility without going to court
4. DNR (do not resuscitate)—Is an order not to attempt cardiopulmonary resuscitation in the event the individual suffers cardiac or respiratory arrest.

NOTE: Violation of DNR order can generate a citation from the State!

5. DNI (do not intubate)—An order not to insert a plastic tube in the throat and into the windpipe to assist with breathing in the event of progressive or impending pulmonary failure.

6. MOLST(medical order for life sustaining treatment) is a document that is a short centralized summary of an individual's treatment preference to ensure transfer of appropriate information among health care providers.
7. FHCDA (family health care decisions act)—When an individual cannot make their own decisions and do not have a health care proxy or legal guardian, FHCDA specifies using a prioritized surrogate list,

Residents with DNR (do not resuscitate) orders should have the following in place:

a. Clear and precise signed DNR order paperwork.
b. A marker on the exterior of the chart.
c. Marker on the resident.
d. MD order.
e. When resident is going out to an appointment or transfer to an acute care setting, a copy of the DNR order must be sent with the accompanying paperwork.
f. Facility must have a clear and precise policy in place on the usage of the hospital DNR in the event of an emergency until the MD can sign the paperwork for a facility DNR

Potential tag: F156—Rights to Refuse Treatment, Experimental Research or to Formulate Advance Directives

Potential tag: F242—Self Determination—Resident's Rights to Make Choices

PHYSICIAN SERVICES

The facility is responsible for ensuring the care of each resident is supervised by a doctor. Every resident must be seen by a doctor at a minimum of every 30 days and the history and physical conduct by the doctor monthly MUST reflect all special needs of the resident e.g. wounds, dialysis, Foleys, colostomy, weight issues, restraints, psychotropic meds etc.

A resident, family/legal representative have the right to know the identity of the primary care doctor in the skilled care facility and how to reach him/her. An alert resident or their family/legal representative have the right to choose to change their primary doctor. Social service department must intervene, and if no reasonable compromise can be reached, the resident has the right to be seen by another doctor in the facility. It must be clearly documented by social services that they intervened and tried to address resident's/representative's concerns before making the change.

Potential tag: F163—right to choose a personal physician

Potential tag: F385—Resident's Care Supervised by a Physician

Potential tag F386—Physician Visits—Review Care/Orders/Notes

Potential tag: F387—Frequency and Timeliness of Physician Visits

Potential tag: F388—Personal (face to face) Visits by Physician, NP or PA

MEDICAL DIRECTOR

Facility must have a doctor who serves as the medical director and is responsible for coordination of medical care and provide guidance and oversight regarding resident care policies.

The role of the Medical Director involves but is not limited to involvement and documentation in the following areas.

a. Accident/Incident investigation reports
b. Supervision of all doctors and the medical unit
c. Development of nosocomial or in house wounds (these should be done on an accident/incident report)
d. Restraint committee meetings
e. Medication errors
f. Review and sign the consultant pharmacist reports
g. Oversight of the resident care policies
h. Ensure that facility is capable of meeting the medical needs of residents admitted, e.g. residents with special needs such as life vests, ventilators, nasogastric tubes etc.
i. Be a member of the quality assessment and assurance committee
j. Present medical concerns at the quality assessment and assurance meetings
k. Aware of effectiveness of x-ray and laboratory services
l. Assist the facility in obtaining contracts with consultants
m. Attend all pharmacy and laboratory meetings
n. Ensure adequate medical coverage to the facility 24/7
o. Must be available to answer calls from the facility if the primary doctor is not available.
p. Ensuring medical staff is providing medical care consistent with current standards or practice
q. Intervening when primary doctor is not addressing acute medical situations
r. Intervening when there are unresolved issues with the primary doctor and residents, families or the interdisciplinary team.

s. Ensuring that nurse practitioners and physician assistants are performing within their scope of practice and the regulatory guidelines.

Potential Tag: F501—Responsibilities of the Medical Director

DISCHARGE/TRANSFER/BEDHOLD

Social Service department must be proactive at informing residents and family/legal representative of the facility's discharge, transfer and bed hold policy upon admission.

Social service involvement precedes admission! Social worker must be involved in ensuring short term care residents can be safely discharged back to the community.

The facility should have discharge/transfer/bed hold forms that are issued to residents/families/legal representative in the event of a discharge from the facility, transfer to another facility or even a therapeutic leave. This form must be signed by the resident/family/legal representative and kept as a part of the resident's medical records.

> All residents transferred or discharged (even to the community) or on therapeutic leave must be given a written copy of the facility's discharge, transfer, and bed hold policy.

> It is advisable to have the resident or family/legal representative sign the form. If this is not possible because of refusal or the nature and time of the transfer, the nurse should write on the form that the resident is unable to or refuses to sign and ensure a copy of the form goes with the resident.

> A copy of the signed form *must* be kept in the resident's medical records.

> After the morning inter-discipline meeting, social services or nursing management should follow up to make sure that all discharged residents were provided with this paperwork.

> It is advisable to keep copies of these forms in a binder in the nursing office for easy access if requested.

When a resident is transferred or discharged from the facility, there must be clear documentation by:

(a) The nurse on the unit and the RN supervisor transferring the resident regarding the reason for the transfer, status of resident when leaving the facility, MD and family notification and the institution resident is transferred to
(b) subsequent documentation by the doctor
(c) social services

All residents transferred to the hospital must have a disposition note entered in the medical records, including the time of admission and the diagnosis.

Every resident must have a clear documented discharge care plan initiated upon admission.

Residents discharged to the community must have paperwork completed by all departments outlining the residents' plan of care, any follow-up required and any teaching.

There must be clear, precise documentation by social services on all discharges regarding the following:

a. Proper placement
b. Community resources, if necessary
c. Support system
d. The phone number and address of any agency responsible for protection and advocacy if necessary
e. Necessary equipment in place e.g. grab bars in showers; wheelchair ramps;

Family notification of any transfers or discharges is extremely important. If the family cannot be reached at the time of transfer/discharge, this must be carried on the 24 hour nursing report until nursing or social services have documented that they were notified.

NOTE: It is important to note that as per The Long Term Care Survey guide, a hospital *cannot* be a final point of discharge. Therefore, even if a resident loses bed hold, a facility cannot make the determination to leave the resident in the hospital. Provision must be made to readmit that resident when a bed becomes available if the hospital is unable to place the resident in another facility.

Potential tag: F157—Notify of Changes

Potential tag: F201—Reasons for Transfer/Discharge of a Resident

Potential tag: F202—Documentation for Transfer/Discharge of a Resident

Potential tag: F203—Notice Requirements before Transfer/Discharge

Potential tag: F204—Preparation for Safe/Orderly Transfer/Discharge

Potential tag: F205—Notice of Bed hold Policy before/upon Transfer

Potential tag: F206—Permitting Resident to Return to the Facility

Potential tag: F250—Provision of Medically Related Social Services

Potential tag F283—Completion of Discharge Summary

Potential tag F284—Post-Discharge Plan of Care

NOTIFICATION OF DOCTOR AND FAMILY

Whenever there is any change to the resident or to the Resident's plan of care, the resident, the doctor and the resident's family/legal representative must be immediately notified and the change must be clearly documented. An alert resident has the right to refuse to have family notified but this must be clearly documented in the medical records.

The name of the person contacted and preferable his or her phone number must be clearly documented in the progress notes also.

If an alert resident refuses to have the family/legal representative notified or there is no legal representative, this must also be clearly documented.

NOTE: The facility must have a system in place for ensuring all contact information on its demographic sheets is accurate!

If nurse is unable to reach the family/legal representative on a particular shift, the information should be carried on the 24 hour nursing report until the family/legal representative is contacted by nursing or social worker.

Family/Legal representative must be notified of:

1. Accidents/incidents
2. Decisions regarding transfers or discharges
3. A change in room or roommate
4. Development of new wounds
5. Weight issues
6. Deterioration in physical, mental or psychological health
7. Need to change a medication or treatment
8. Start or end of therapy
9. Any scheduled consults, especially those outside the facility
10. Need for wander bracelet

11. Thickened liquids or fluid restrictions
12. Any other changes in the facility impacting on the resident

Potential tag: F157—Resident/Family/Legal Representative Notification of Changes

RESIDENT'S PERSONAL ROPERTY

Residents have the right to be free from misappropriation of their properties

As per the New York State Operation Manual, misappropriation of resident's property means the deliberate misplacement, exploitation or wrongful temporary or permanent use of a resident's belongings or money without the resident's consent. To ensure accountability when dealing with resident's property, the following is best practice:

1. All of a resident's property should be clearly labeled to prevent misplacement.
2. All property needs to be logged on a property sheet, including clothing, shoes, belts, electronics, glasses, hearing aids.
3. If a resident refuses to have items labeled, a nursing note and a care plan must be implemented. Social services must also be informed so they can provide counseling to the resident and family/legal representative in the event items are misplaced.
4. If the resident is admitted with items that are not properly logged and they are misplaced, it is that resident's word against the facility as to whether or not items are missing.
5. When residents are transferred to the hospital or during room change, the facility must have a system in place for ensuring all the resident's possessions are secured.
6. When family brings in items along the way, these must be added to the property sheet.
7. Facility must have some system in place for residents to obtain a locked drawer or closet to store their valuables.
8. Facility must have a system in place to ensure that all of the resident's clothing is safely returned after laundry.
9. All residents' report of missing property must be investigated and a resolution reached.

Potential tag: F224—Prohibit Mistreatment, Neglect/Misappropriation

THERAPEUTIC ACTIVITIES

Recreation and social interactions are extremely important in maintaining the quality of life. When life's daily tasks of cooking, cleaning, paying bills, raising children no longer take up the bulk of the day, it is essential to fill that time with something less constructive but meaningful.

Therapeutic recreation provides our residents with a daily purpose and fosters socialization with their peers. Part of the ongoing assessment of residents is to identify what activities they enjoyed in their leisure time and strive to maintain some similarity.

Resident council meetings offer residents their right to meet as a group and voice their concerns and complaints to the interdisciplinary team.

1. The recreation department must have structured and meaningful activities that residents enjoy partaking in.
2. A comprehensive recreation assessment must be completed on every resident and their desires clearly documented so the interdisciplinary team is aware.
3. When the recreation department puts interventions in place, these must be assessed for the role of nursing. E.g., recreation putting an intervention that a resident enjoys rock music must be clearly written on the certified nursing assistant accountability record so they are aware of this daily and can ensure that need is met.
4. It is also recommended that recreation department leave some recreational items (e.g., cards, crossword puzzles, artwork, etc.) in a secure location in the dayroom or nursing station so nursing can ensure continued therapeutic recreation while residents are out of recreational programs or ensure entertaining television programs that appeal to the residents.
5. Activity calendar must be clearly posted on units and other highly visualized areas.

6. Recreation department needs to provide nursing department with a copy of all resident council minutes after each meeting so the director of nursing/designee can review for any reported instances of abuse, neglect, or mistreatment.
7. **NOTE:** It is advisable for the director of nursing/designee and other department heads to attend resident council meetings.
8. **NOTE:** The residents' concerns and complaints should be everyone's concern!
9. Nursing department should provide recreation department with an updated list of the diabetics and the residents on thickened liquids.

Potential tag: F242—Self Determination—Residents Right to Make Choices

Potential tag: F244—Listen/Act on Group Grievance Recommendations

Potential tag: F245—Resident Participates in Activities

Potential tag: F248—Activities Programs Meet Individual Needs

SMOKING

For facilities that permit smoking, provision must be made to ensure residents' right to smoke is honored in a safe manner.

EVERY resident admitted to the facility must be assessed and documented whether they are a smoker or not.

If the resident is NOT a smoker no follow-up assessment is required.

If the resident is deemed a smoker or has history of smoking, a comprehensive assessment must be completed by the interdisciplinary team of doctor, nurse, recreation and social work.

A smoking contract must be signed with the resident clearly delineating the facility's smoking policy and consequences of not complying with same.

A resident identified as a smoker and wishes to smoke must be fully assessed for safety including but not limited to:

a). Dexterity to safely light and hold cigarettes.
b). Can resident safely use ash tray.
c). Need for a smoking apron.
d). Does resident allow cigarette to burn to the butt and resulting in burns to the fingers
e). Need for smoking fire retardant glove or cigarette holder
f). Not pocketing lit cigarettes
g). Not eating cigarette butts
h). Not sharing cigarettes with other residents

All smoking rooms must have a fire retardant smoking blanket readily available in the room.

Smoking sessions must be supervised by designated staff at all times.

There should be a wide range of smoking times to minimize non-compliance with the smoking rules.

The facility's smoking room must have a proper approved ventilation system.

NOTE: For facilities that do not have a smoking room and residents smoke outside, must have a policy and plan in place for inclement weather!

Facility MUST keep all resident smoking paraphernalia securely locked in a metal receptacle and provide same to resident at smoking times.

The smoking assessment must be done:

1. Every three months
2. When any significant changes occur
3. Changes in activities of daily living
4. Cognitive changes

NOTE: If an alert resident on oxygen choses to smoke, the facility cannot prevent the resident from smoking. However, UNDER no circumstances can the resident take the oxygen near the smoking room. However, resident and family/legal representative teaching and encouragement should be provided regarding smoking cessation options.

NOTE: It is important for families/legal representatives to be aware of the facility's smoking policy and to give all smoking paraphernalia to staff.

Potential tag: F 280—Right to Participate in Care Planning

WEIGHT MANAGEMENT

The management of nutrition in skilled care facility residents involves an interdisciplinary approach starting from admission. The comprehensive clinical assessment and the dietary assessment provide pertinent information regarding actual or potential impaired nutrition and weight management.

Many factors affect nutrition including but not limited to chewing and swallowing issues, medications and comorbidities. Appetite can be affected by the appearance of the food, resident's choices and the dining environment. In an effort to effectively manage residents weights and address any actual or potential unplanned weight gain or lost, the following is best practice:

>The admission nurse must ensure that all admissions/re-admissions are weighed and measured and the weight and height are entered on the admission sheet. If the resident refuses, the refusal must be documented on the twenty-four-hour nursing report so the morning shift can follow up.

>Remind the admission nurse to add the names of all admissions and readmissions on the weekly and monthly weight sheets.

>All new admissions/readmissions must be weighed weekly for the first four weeks then monthly thereafter. It may be necessary to continue weekly weights if a resident is unstable.

>It is advisable that monthly weights on all residents be completed by at least the fifth of the month.

>When reviewing monthly weights, it is advisable to review weights for the current month and the past two months so you are looking at three months weights and can clearly identify any trends. This should be done with the dietitian and nurse

together. All weekly weights obtained should be reviewed at this time also.

Weekly weight list must be adjusted after monthly weight meetings.

Weight notes must be written by the interdisciplinary team—dietitian, nurse, and the doctor. The nurse and dietitian can write together and then leave a copy of the notes for the doctor if he/she is not readily available.

When addressing a resident with significant weight lost, every intervention and/or effort to maintain resident's ability for oral intake must be clearly documented.

The dietitian looks at weight in terms of (a) calories, (b) meal and supplement intake, (c) swallowing or chewing abnormalities (d) resident preference

Nursing looks at weight in terms of (a) acute conditions—e.g., antibiotic therapy, edema; (b) intake of meals and supplements; (c) consults; psychiatry, psychosocial issues—e.g. death of a spouse; history of depression, etc. (d) co-morbidities, .e.g. failure to thrive, cancer, hypo or hyperthyroidism (f) oral conditions.

The doctor looks at weight in terms of (a) medications review—e.g., changing of Celexa to Remeron, need for appetite stimulants; and (b) clinical workup in terms of labs and/or consults (c) side effects of medications

Dietitians look at weights in terms of percentage; nurses, in pounds. Therefore, the following require documentation:

a. For residents under one hundred pounds, *three* or more pounds lost/gained
b. Residents over one hundred pounds, *five* or more pounds lost/gained

c. Even when they don't meet the aforementioned, any resident's weight showing a trending up or down over the three months should be addressed.

Significant weight loss or gain should be documented as

a). avoidable or unavoidable
b). Beneficial or undesirable
c). Relation to resident's usual body weight
d). With weight gain always mention absence or presence of edema, ascites, shortness of breath, moist cough to rule out underlying congestive heart failure

Dialysis residents with significant weight gain or loss should not be just attributed to fluctuation as a result of dialysis. A full investigation must be done and interdisciplinary documentation must be in place.

Certified nursing assistants should not write the weights directly on the weight book or enter on electronic medical record. This must be done by a nurse only.

Remind the certified nursing assistants to weigh residents in a consistent manner—e.g., same scale, without excessive clothing, with splints removed, with wheelchair weights subtracted and to re-weigh residents who show loss or gain of 3 or more pounds than the last weight, preferably with the nurse's supervision.

Significant weight loss or gain should be shared with the MDS coordinator to determine if resident requires a significant change.

NOTE: Facility must ensure that it has a system in place for residents to receive adequate hydration. E.g. Labelled cup of water at bedside daily or a central hydration station with a schedule for distribution! Issues of weight gain or loss could be determined by making reference to the resident's height and the resident's recommended ideal body weight (IBW) or the resident's usual body weight (UBW).

MDS must reflect weight and address any weight loss or gain.

Care plan must be completed.

Potential tag: F150—Resident's Rights (as it relates to food preference)

Potential tag: F272—Comprehensive Assessment

Potential tag: F279—Comprehensive Care Plan

Potential tag: F280—Comprehensive Care Plan Revision

Potential tag: F282—Qualified Services in Accordance with Care Plan

Potential tag: F325—Maintain Nutritional Status, unless Unavoidable

Potential tag: F327—Provide Residents with Sufficient Fluid to Maintain Hydration

Potential tag: F329—Drug Regimen is Free from Unnecessary Drugs

Potential tag: F361—Qualified Dietitian—Director of Food Services

Potential tag: F385—Resident's Care Supervised by a Physician

Potential tag: F501—Responsibilities of the Medical Director

Potential tag: F520—Quality Assessment and Assurance

DINING OBSERVATION

The dining environment, the supervision residents need from staff, the smell and appearance of meals and resident choices can significantly impact on appetite which is essential for weight management. Each resident should be properly assessed for the amount of assistance required with feeding to ensure adequate help is received. During meal times,

All TV MUST be turned off and music can be turned on.

Staff members are encouraged to interact with the residents while assisting them.

All nursing staff must be on their respective units at mealtimes. Staff breaks and lunchtimes should not be scheduled during resident mealtimes.

There must be a seating arrangement chart that is drawn up by nursing and dietary departments and should be updated at least monthly.

Dietitian should ensure that the kitchen is aware of this seating arrangement to ensure that the food truck is stacked accordingly.

When making a seating arrangement chart, staff must be mindful of residents on special diets but will take food from peers' trays!

Staff should serve one table at a time completely before moving on to another table.

All residents entering the dining room must have their hands clean with Sani Wipes, even the latecomers.

A nurse must be present in the dining room for all meals.

All nurses must close medication and treatment carts during mealtime and assist. One must be in the dining room and one must walk the halls to monitor residents eating in their rooms.

Staff must make sure the suction machine is uncovered and functional for each meal.

Residents requiring finger-sticks before meals must have that done in privacy before being wheeled into the dining room.

Recreation and rehab departments should be aware of when meals are being served so residents can be back on respective units on time to allow for proper setup at mealtimes.

Resident should be offered clothing protectors.

 Residents that require total assistance with feeding must be seated together.

Staff should be seated when feeding residents—Dignity!

As much as possible staff should avoid mixing food items in order not to make the food unpalatable and unattractive, unless it is resident's preference to do so.

All residents who are on NPO (nothing by mouth) should be removed from the dining rooms at mealtimes.

Facility must have a log to record how much each resident consumed for every meal. It is advisable to have this in one binder for all residents for easy documentation at mealtimes.

Ensure that nursing staff is not serving supplements such as Ensure with meals, as this will minimize intake of meal.

Feeders' trays should *not* be opened before a staff member is ready to feed them.

Nursing staff should be mindful to order the alternate or substitute meal for a resident as per preference or after observing that a resident is not consuming current meal.

Dietary needs requires an interdisciplinary approach from nursing and dietary. Nursing staff should be aware of residents' diets and special needs such as those receiving double portions or requiring special utensils etc.

Dietary must be mindful of the times that meals are served as there must be no more than 14 hours between supper in the evening and breakfast in the morning!

Remind staff *not* to put dirty trays back on the food truck while other residents' meals are still on the truck.

Kitchen should do a second sweep after each mealtime to ensure that all soiled dishes are removed from the units.

NOTE: Residents that require assistive devices at mealtimes such as built up spoon or scoop dish involve the coordination of the dietary department and the rehab department.

NOTE: It is very important for the facility to have a food committee comprised of residents to allow for feedback on whether the food is palatable, attractive and served at the right temperature.

NOTE: Menus must be generated daily and made readily available to residents either by delivering them to the residents or posted same in a highly visualized place and at residents' eye level.

NOTE: Dietary must ensure there is adequate amount of snacks on the units to be provided per doctor's order, per residents' request and for diabetics at bedtime or early morning as needed.

NOTE: It is very important for all diets to have a doctor's order and to be documented on the certified nursing assistant accountability records so that the certified nursing assistants are fully aware of diet consistencies and diet changes as they are the key personnel at mealtimes.

NOTE: If a facility utilizes feeding assistants as defined by the State's law, they must be trained to call for the nurse in emergency situations and they should feed only residents who have no complicated feeding problems.

Potential tag: F240—Care and Environment Promotes Quality of Life

Potential tag: F241—Dignity and Respect of Individuality

Potential tag: F360—Diet Meets Needs of Each Resident.

Potential tag: F361-Employment of a Qualified Dietitian

Potential tag: F363—Menu Meets Residents Needs

Potential tag: F364—Food is Palatable, Attractive and at Right Temperature

Potential tag: F365--Food must be in Form to Meet Individual Needs

Potential tag: F366—Substitutes of Similar Nutritive Value

Potential tag: F367—Therapeutic Diet Prescribed by the Doctor

Potential tag F368—Frequency of Meals/Snacks at Bedtime

Potential tag F369—Assistive Devices/Eating Equipment and Utensils

Potential tag: F373—Proper Usage and Documentation of Paid Feeding Assistants

RESIDENTS WITH NASOGASTRIC AND GASTROSTOMY TUBES

The decision to insert a feeding tube to attain or maintain a resident's nutritional status may be necessary. There must be clear and concise documentation of resident, family/legal representative notification and consent to the procedure. Every attempt made to maintain the resident's nutritional status through oral intake must also be well documented. If a resident is admitted with a feeding tube or had it inserted while a resident in the facility, the following is best practice:

It is not recommended that a resident with a nasogastric tube (NG) be in a long-term facility for longer than a week, secondary to the high risk for aspiration pneumonia.

All feeding tube orders must have a clear reason for usage. Most of the times, a feeding tube is ordered due to dysphagia or aspiration.

If the feeding tube is inserted after the resident is admitted to the facility, there must be clear, concise interdisciplinary documentation indicating that ALL other options have been explored before resorting to a feeding tube—in other words feeding tube usage was unavoidable!

Make sure there is documentation of the family's involvement.

When a resident's gastrostomy dislodges, it is advisable to do an accident/incident report and conduct an investigation to rule out abuse or mistreatment.

Residents should be fed overnight to free them up to attend activities during the day hours.

Facility must have a policy in place for checking for gastrostomy placement prior to start of feeding and after an acute episode of vomiting.

Bolus feeding should be considered for residents who are refusing to allow the full time for formula to run and for those residents that are constantly pulling out the feeding tube.

NOTE: Nursing/Dietary must monitor resident for complications related to the tube feed. E.g. diarrhea. May have to consider changing the rate of administration or the type of formula.

If an abdominal binder is necessary, it should be care planned for and treated as a restraint.

Orders for feeding tube should clearly state the following:

a. Name of Resident
b. Start time (preferable 5:00–6:00 p.m.)
c. Formula
d. Amount to be administered
e. Flow rate
f. End time
g. Diagnosis

The tube feeding bag and the flush system *must* be clearly labeled with the resident's name and the date. The bag must be changed every twenty-four hours.

Certified nursing assistant accountability record must indicate that the resident is a tube feeder and nothing by mouth (NPO). The instructions to keep head of bed elevated thirty-five to forty-five degrees must also be included on the certified nursing assistant accountability record.

Certified nursing assistant must be instructed not to turn off feeding tube during care.

Every attempt should be made to maintain a resident's oral status. Resident can have tube feedings and oral snacks.

There must be an order for cleaning the gastrostomy site and the treatment written on the treatment administration record.

MDS must reflected same

Care plan must be in place.

A dislodged gastrostomy can be re-inserted by an RN. However, this protocol must be clearly stated in the facility's policy.

Surveyors often check the following:

1. Reason for insertion of feeding tube and need for continued usage
2. Interventions that were in place prior to feeding tube placement
3. Appropriate labeling of the formula, tubing and flush set up.
4. Flush schedule
5. Meds are not crushed and mixed together
6. If resident receives oral recreational snacks are same provided?
7. Flush is done after each medication *and* before and after the entire medication administration based on the particular resident per doctor's order (e.g., resident at risk for congestive heart failure should have schedule for less fluid)
8. Medications are allowed to run in by gravity
9. Compliance with start and end times
10. Proper elevation of resident's head
11. Excessive weight loss or gain (feeding needs to be adjusted by doctor/dietitian)
12. Pump and pole are clear
13. Proper technique and infection control when hanging the feeding or giving meds
14. Proper nursing technique during med administration via feeding tube

Potential tag: F272—Comprehensive Assessment

Potential tag: F279—Comprehensive Care Plan

Potential tag: F280—Comprehensive Care Plan Revision

Potential tag: F282—Qualified Services in Accordance with Care Plan

Potential tag: F321—Resident who is able to eat enough with Assistance is not fed by a GT

Potential tag: F322--NG treatment/Services—Restore Eating Skills

Potential tag: F325—Maintain Nutritional Status Unless Unavoidable

Potential tag: F327—Sufficient Fluid to Maintain Hydration

Potential tag: F328—Treatment/Care for Special Care Needs

Potential tag: F385—Resident's Care Supervised by a Physician

Potential tag: F441—Infection Control (During Med Pass)

Potential tag: F501—Responsibilities of the Medical Director

RESIDENTS ON THICKENED
LIQUIDS AND SPECIAL DIETS

Many medical conditions impact on a resident's eating, chewing and swallowing functions causing coughing and choking during meal consumption. Some of these may be acute, e.g. oral and dental conditions, and others chronic such as strokes or aging. Residents on thickened liquid are at high risk for dehydration and should be closely monitored.

As per the New York State Department of Health Nursing Home Incident Reporting Manual,

   a. If a resident is served or manages to obtain food of incorrect consistency and chokes and requires staff intervention this is reportable.
   b. If the resident requires thickened liquids and was served or managed to obtain incorrect consistency and choked and required staff intervention this is reportable.
   c. Choking incidents are reportable to the Department of Health.

. When making a seating arrangement chart, staff must be mindful of residents on special diets who may be willing to take food from peers' trays.

. It is very important for the recreation department and café staff (if there is one on site) to be aware of residents on thickened liquids or special diets. The list must be updated as changes are made.

. Thickened liquid order MUST be written on the medication administration record so that nurses giving fluids with medications are aware of this.

. It is important that doctors' orders for diet or fluid consistency change are documented on the certified nursing assistant accountability record.

. It is important that family/legal representative is aware of the resident's diet.

. Whenever a resident has an episode of choking, the resident must be assessed by nursing, medical, dietary and speech therapist and the assessments must be documented in the resident's medical records.

. It is advisable to do an accident/incident report and conduct an investigation for all instances of choking.

NOTE: If a facility utilizes feeding assistants as defined by the State's law, they must be trained to call for the nurse in emergency situations and they should feed only residents who have no complicated feeding problems.

NOTE: As Per the New York State Nursing Home Reporting Manual, all choking incidents are reportable to the State!

Potential tag: F272—Comprehensive Assessment

Potential tag: F279—Comprehensive Care Plan

Potential tag: F280—Comprehensive Care Plan Revision

Potential tag: F282—Qualified Services in Accordance with Care Plan

Potential tag F323—Free of Accidents, Hazards/Supervision/Devices

Potential tag: F385—Resident's Care Supervised by a Physician (Must be on the monthly H&P)

FLUID RESTRICTIONS

Residents with certain medical conditions require fluid restrictions, e.g. residents with congestive heart failure and residents receiving dialysis.

The facility must have a system in place for recording the fluid intake and output of these residents. Residents on fluid restrictions must be monitored for compliance or non-compliance. Non-compliance could be taking less or taking more than the recommended amount. The following is best when monitoring residents with fluid restrictions:

1. Residents on fluid restrictions need a doctor's order for the amount of fluid that should be given within 24 hours and why the resident requires the restriction.
2. Dietitian must have clear documentation in the progress notes on why resident is on fluid restriction.
3. The dietitian must have a sheet that clearly breaks down how much fluid resident is supposed to receive on each shift.
4. The fluid breakdown sheet must clearly reflect how much fluid is provided by dietary with meals and how much fluid should be given by nursing.
5. To ensure that it is not missed by nurses, the fluid restriction should also be written on the medication administration record with a directive to see the breakdown sheet.
6. Fluid restriction must be clearly written on the certified nursing assistant accountability records by the nurse.
7. Residents with fluid restrictions require documented monitoring of their intake and out-put.
8. If a resident is taking less than the recommended fluid restriction, there is a high risk for dehydration and this must be addressed with the doctor promptly.
9. If the resident is taking more than the recommended fluid restriction, there is the potential for fluid overload and can lead to complications such as congestive heart failure and this must also be addressed with the doctor promptly.

10. The doctor, dietitian and nurse should have documentations in the progress notes.
11. There must be documented ongoing teaching to non-compliant residents.
12. Because of the risk for dehydration, the doctor should have a system in place for monitoring labs periodically and nurses should be assessing for physical signs of dehydration such as dry skin and mucus membranes.
13. Recreation staff and the café staff should be aware of residents on fluid restrictions. The list must be updated as changes are made.

Care plan must be completed.

MDS must reflect diagnosis.

Potential tag: F272—Comprehensive Assessment

Potential tag: F279—Comprehensive Care Plan

Potential tag: F280—Comprehensive Care Plan Revision

Potential tag: F282—Qualified Services in Accordance with Care Plan

Potential tag: F327—Sufficient Fluid to Maintain Hydration

Potential tag: F385—Resident's Care Supervised by a Physician (Must be on the monthly history and physical)

RESIDENT WITH DIALYSIS NEEDS

Dialysis is a treatment that does some of the things done by healthy kidneys. There are two types of dialysis:

a). Peritoneal dialysis
b). Hemodialysis.

Peritoneal dialysis is done by inserting dialysate fluid through a catheter in the stomach and then draining after a few hours.

Hemodialysis is a process that uses a machine with a special filter that functions like an artificial kidney to clean the blood as the kidneys can no longer perform this function due to chronic kidney disease. To get the blood into the dialyzer, surgical access is gained through the arm or upper chest wall by an AV shunt, fistula or Perma-catheter.

As part of the Medicare/Medicaid survey process to nursing homes, a sample of dialysis residents records are reviewed. The following is considered best practice to ensure quality care:

. The facility must have a signed contract with the dialysis center.

- The doctor's order must reflect (a) the days of the week and the time; (b) the name of center with its phone number; (c) the transportation company with its phone number; (d) the type of access—e.g., AV shunt, fistula or Perma-catheter—and location; and (e) the doctor's order for any emergency, such as bleeding, signs and symptoms of infection and monitoring for bruit and thrill accordingly. Note: Bruit and thrill are only checked with AV shunt and fistula.
- Make sure that all doctor's orders for medications and treatments are accounted for before the resident goes to dialysis or after the resident returns from dialysis. The facility cannot record "on hold" or "out on pass" for medications when the resident is at dialysis.

- For residents receiving medications at the dialysis center, the doctor's order and the medication administration record need to clearly reflect this.
- **NOTE**: On every monthly progress note, the doctor must mention resident is on dialysis.
- A nursing note *must* be written pre- and post-dialysis with the weight, blood pressure, pulse and temperature. The post dialysis note must indicate how the shunt or fistula site looks and the resident must be monitored for bleeding and bruit and thrill accordingly.
- The nurses must sign their entry in the dialysis communication book pre-dialysis and the receiving nurse upon return from dialysis must review and initial dialysis center communication and follow-up with any orders/recommendations with the doctor as needed.
- It is advisable to have clear signs in resident's record not to draw blood or take blood pressure on the affected side. It's very important for an outside lab technician to know this also.
- All dialysis residents must have a notebook that goes with them to the dialysis center for communication between your facility and the dialysis center.
- It is advisable to put a line down the center of each page in these books and label one side with your facility name and the other side with the dialysis center name so it is clear who is communicating what.

Sunshine Center for Rehabilitation	Waterfront Dialysis Center

. If the resident is sent to the hospital from the dialysis center, the RN supervisor on duty must notify the doctor and family/legal representative and document this in the medical records.

- The certified nursing assistants accountability record must clearly state the following:

  a. The days the resident goes to dialysis
  b. The pickup time
  c. Report to nurse of any bleeding, swelling, redness at the site or complaint of pain
  d. Fluid restrictions, if recommended by the dietitian

- Dietary must be aware of all dialysis residents and their pickup time so they can prepare bagged meals accordingly.
- Even though some weight fluctuations are expected, this must be clearly documented in the dietitian notes.
- If the weight fluctuation is significant (as determined by the facility policy, generally over five pounds), interdisciplinary documentation by the dietician, doctor, and nurse is encouraged to rule out other factors that may be affecting the weight.
- MDS must reflect resident is on dialysis.
- Care plan must be completed.

Potential tag: F272—Comprehensive Assessment

Potential tag: F279—Comprehensive Care Plan

Potential tag: F280—Comprehensive Care Plan Revision

Potential tag: F282—Qualified Services in Accordance with Care Plan

Potential tag: F309—Provide care/services for highest well-being

Potential tag F385—Resident's Care Supervised by a Physician (Must be carried on monthly history and physical)

Potential tag: F441—Infection Control

Potential tag: F500—Use of Outside Professional Resources

INDWELLING CATHETERS—FOLEY, SUPRAPUBIC AND UROSTOMY

The regulation surrounding the use of indwelling catheters focuses on whether there is a clear clinical reason for insertion and whether there is a clear clinical reason for maintaining it.

The plan of care must be properly implemented and documented by various shifts.

Proper infection control techniques must be used to minimize infection. In an effort to avoid unnecessary prolonged used of an indwelling catheter, there must be ongoing assessments.

- When a resident has a Foley, suprapubic or urostomy catheter (upon admission or inserted in-house), the doctor's order must clearly state the following:

  a. The size
  b. Daily catheter care method
  c. Change schedule (which is often monthly if it is for long-term usage)
  d. The flush schedule (decision of the doctor)

- When a resident is admitted with a *Foley* catheter, if there is no clear medical reason for its usage, it is advisable for the doctor to give an order for removal and for the resident to be monitored for voiding. Observations must be documented on the twenty-four-hour nursing report.
- Clear medical reasons could be any of the following:

  a. Urinary retention
  b. Neurogenic bladder
  c. Bladder cancer
  d. BPH

e. Urethral stricture
f. Obstructive uropathy
g. Stage 3 sacral ulcer (to prevent worsening but not for long-term use)
h. Stage 4 sacral ulcer

- Suprapubic and urostomy catheters are often used as last option, therefore, they are not to be removed unless there are written directions from an urologist.
- On each monthly visit, the doctor *must* clearly document on the catheter and the medical reason for continued usage. The notes must include attempts made to remove the catheter.
- If a resident with a permanent catheter has developed a urinary tract infection more than once, the doctor must put interventions in place to prevent recurrence—e.g., extra fluids, cranberry tablets or long term prophalactic antibiotic usage.
- A resident with a permanent catheter should be followed with an urologist appointment at the minimum of every six months.
- Residents with urinary catheters should be assessed for pain.
- For residents with suprapubic catheters, the catheter can be changed by an RN in-house. Some facilities are more comfortable with having the urologist change them. If it is done by the RN, the facility's policy must reflect the same.
- If a resident's catheter is dislodged, it is highly recommended that an accident/incident report be made out and that an investigation be conducted to rule out abuse, neglect, or mistreatment.
- Nurse must notify the doctor of decreased output or changes in urine color and consistency—e.g., bloody, cloudy.
- If a catheter is removed per a doctor's order, resident's name should be placed on the twenty-four-hour nursing report for monitoring for adequate urine output at a minimum of 72 hours.
- Change schedule must be written on the treatment administration record and boxed off so that nurse can sign for it. A flush schedule must also be made out.
- To prevent infection, staff should ensure that the catheter tubing and/or bag are never put on the floor.

- Staff must monitor the labia, penis or scrotum for any openings secondary to ongoing pressure from the catheter.
- All drainage bags must be covered for privacy and kept below the level of the waist, in or out of bed. If resident refuses, this must be care-planned.
- To ensure that output is recorded every shift, it is advisable that all residents with catheters stay on the twenty-four-hour nursing report to ensure output is charted in the resident's progress notes every shift. Only one line needs to be recorded, unless there are other acute changes: "Output is ——— ccs" or they can be carried on the treatment administration record.
- The daily assignment sheet made out for each shift by the charge nurses must mention all residents with catheters so that the certified nursing assistants can document the output.
- The certified nursing assistant accountability record must also state that the resident has a catheter.
- Daily catheter care needs to be documented on the certified nursing assistant accountability record.
- The nurse must remind certified nursing assistants to inform nurse of changes such as decrease urinary output, cloudy or bloody urine.
- If the facility uses leg bags, the schedule for changing to leg bag when out of bed and then back to drainage bag when in bed must be on the certified nursing assistant accountability record.
- When leg bags should be stored in a tied plastic bag when not in use must be stated.
- Anchor the catheter to avoid excessive tugging on it during transfer and care.
- Catheter must be captured on the MDS.
- Care plan must be completed.

Potential tag: F157—Family Notification of Change

Potential tag: F241—Dignity (keep bag covered and minimize embarrassment)

Potential tag: F272—Comprehensive Assessment

Potential tag: F279—Comprehensive Care Plan

Potential tag: F280—Comprehensive Care Plan Revision

Potential tag F281—Services are provided to Meet Professional Standard

Potential tag: F312—ADL Care for Dependent Residents

Potential tag: F315—No catheter; prevent UTI; restore bladder

Potential tag: F327—Resident is Receiving Sufficient Fluid for Hydration

Potential tag F328—Treatment/Care for Special Needs

Potential tag: F385—Resident's Care Supervised by a Physician (must be carried on the monthly history and physical)

Potential tag: F441—Infection Control

Potential tag: F498—Proficiency of Nursing Aides

COLOSTOMY AND ILEOSTOMY CARE

A colostomy is a surgical opening in the abdomen through which a piece of the colon (large intestine) is diverted.

An ileostomy is a surgical opening in the abdomen through which a piece of the ileum (small intestine) is diverted.

These openings allow for excrement of fecal matter into an attached bag. These procedures are created to bypass a damaged portion of the colon. Staff should be aware that:

The doctor's order must state:

    a. size
    b. diagnosis
    c. How often care is provided

Change colostomy wafer every seventy-two hours, and change the bag as needed.

If there is excoriation at the site, the doctor must be notified and there must be an order for treatment.

The wafer must be changed by a nurse who must assess the site.

The daily bag change is done by the nursing assistant, based on facility protocol.

Colostomy and ileostomy must be documented on the treatment administration record and the certified nursing assistant accountability record.

Staff must be very mindful of the fact that these residents have issues with dignity and they must ensure that the attached bag is properly secured to prevent leakage.

Bags must be changed in a timely manner to prevent over filling.

Staff must be educated concerning stool consistency difference, based on the type of ostomy.

Ostomy must be clearly reflected on the doctor monthly progress notes.

MDS must reflect ostomy.

Care plan must be completed.

Potential tag: F241—Dignity (keep bag covered and minimize embarrassment)

Potential tag: F272—Comprehensive Assessment

Potential tag: F279—Comprehensive Care Plan

Potential tag: F280—Comprehensive Care Plan Revision

Potential tag F281—Services are provided to Meet Professional Standard

Potential tag: F312—ADL Care for Dependent Residents

Potential tag: F315—No catheter; prevent UTI; restore bladder

Potential tag: F327—Resident is Receiving Sufficient Fluid for Hydration

Potential tag F328—Treatment/Care for Special Needs

Potential tag: F385—Resident's Care Supervised by a Physician (must be on the monthly history and physical)

Potential tag: F441—Infection Control

Potential tag: F498—Proficiency of Nursing Aides

OXYGEN THERAPY

Residents with certain medical conditions require oxygen therapy e.g. asthma, chronic pulmonary obstructive disease. Residents may require it continuously or as needed.

Because of the combustible nature of oxygen, usage and storage must be properly regulated in the facility. Facility should ensure the following:

Oxygen therapy requires a doctor's order stating

    a. how many liters/min
    b. Frequency (continuous or prn)
    c. Route (nasal cannula or face mask)

For residents on continuous oxygen, it is advisable to have container of sterile water attached to the concentrator for humidification.

NOTE: All residents on oxygen (standard or PRN) must have a sign on their room door indicating "Oxygen Usage"

Oxygen must be documented on the treatment administration record and the certified nursing assistant accountability record.

All oxygen tubing must be dated and changed at least weekly per facility's policy.

It is advisable to attach a small plastic bag to the concentrator in which the tubing is stored when not in use, for infection control. (**NOTE:** This should be done for other tubing).

NOTE: If an alert resident on oxygen chooses to smoke, the facility cannot block resident from smoking. However, resident should *not* be permitted to take the oxygen tank to the smoking area secondary to potential for harm to self and others.

There must be clear interdisciplinary documentation on resident teaching and the doctor's attempts to offer patches to assist with smoking cessation.

NOTE: Provisions for sufficient oxygen must be made for residents on continuous oxygen therapy when going for appointments.

Facilities must put protocols in place to empower RN to initiate oxygen therapy on emergency basis and later obtain doctor's ratification order.

All tanks *must* be stored in a holder.

Care Plan must be completed

MDS must reflect Oxygen Usage.

Potential tag: F441—Infection Control

Potential tag: 323—Free of Accidents/Hazards

TRACHEOSTOMY AND VENTILATOR USAGE

A tracheostomy is an opening in the throat to aid breathing. A ventilator is a machine connected to a breathing tube which connects to the body via the nose, the mouth or a tracheostomy. It is used to help residents that are having difficulty breathing on their own.

For a resident with a tracheostomy, speech is severely impaired secondary to the lack of air flowing over the vocal cords which is an essential component for speech. These residents often communicate by covering the tracheal opening with a finger or may have an order from the doctor for a speaking valve as part of the weaning period.

NOTE: Residents covering the tracheostomy with their finger or hand are at increased risk for infection. It is advisable that doctors assess tracheostomy residents for speaking valve if they are able to tolerate.

The speaking valve is a device that fits on the end of the trachea and forces air upwards through the normal voice box, nostril or mouth routes and allow for speech sounds.

NOTE: These residents utilize oxygen. ALL residents that utilize oxygen must have the oxygen signage on the door; "Oxygen in Use. No Smoking".

Tracheostomy Care:

1. Must have doctor's order for:
    a. Shirley or inner cannula size
    b. Oxygen usage
    c. Frequency of suctioning
    d. Treatment to tracheostomy site
    e. Frequency for inner cannula change
    f. Frequency for tracheostomy collar tie change
    g. Frequency for use of a speaking valve

2. Ensure there is an extra inner cannula readily available at the resident's bedside. It is advisable to have THREE cannulas. One the current size, one smaller size and one bigger size.
3. The suction machine must be clean and in proper working order in the event of an emergency.
4. These residents should be monitored on every half hour rounds at a minimum.
5. An ambu bag MUST be present at the resident's bed side.
6. All necessary supplies including gauge, ties, inner cannula, saline squirts should be readily available at bedside.
7. The doctor must be promptly notified of excessive secretions and any foul smelling secretions.
8. If resident is a male, ensure that there are no excessive facial hair or beard secondary to the risk for infection.
9. Ensure that the ties securing the trache are not too tight to avoid pressure that can lead to ulceration.
10. Monitor the skin around the tracheal opening every shift for breakdown or signs of infection.
11. Tubing not in use should be stored in a plastic bag for infection control.
12. Ensure proper humidification of oxygen to prevent nasal drying.
13. The doctor must document his observations on the resident's tracheostomy on his monthly progress notes.
14. The tracheostomy site must be clean and dry.
15. The certified nursing accountability record should indicate that the resident has a tracheostomy and directions to report any respiratory distress to nurse or respiratory therapist promptly.
16. **NOTE:** If resident eats by mouth, he or she must be very closely supervised at meal times.
17. All tracheostomies must be carried on the treatment administration record. The treatment record needs to reflect the components of the order listed above.
18. If speaking valve is used it is cleansed by washing in warm soapy water daily, rinsing under tap water and allowing to air dry. Speaking valves should also be documented on the treatment administration record and the certified nursing assistant record.

Ventilators:

NOTE: Staff should be trained to respond to all alarms promptly!

Residents on ventilators must have the following doctor's order in place:

a. Ventilator Settings
b. Oxygen Usage
c. Any weaning from the ventilator
d. Usage of a speaking valve
e. Size of the Shirley (inner cannula)
f. Frequency of suctioning
g. Tracheostomy care

Certified nursing assistants should be taught not to disconnect the tubing during care.

Mouth care is extremely important. Nursing assistants must report any excessive secretions.

A ventilator unit, must have functional alarms that are audible in the nursing stations and in the hallways.

NOTE: Facility must have system and a log in place for ensuring all machines are properly maintained.

NOTE: For residents who are ventilator dependent, it is advisable for the respiratory therapists to document the resident's status every shift. E.g. any treatments administered and outcome; description of secretions; rule out signs and symptoms of infection.

All ventilators must be carried on treatment administration record. The treatment administration record must reflect all components of the order.

All ventilators must be documented on the certified nursing assistant record and with clear instructions to report any shortness of breath promptly to the nurse or respiratory therapist.

NOTE: Most of these residents are immunocompromised and are at risk for skin breakdown Facility must be very proactive!

NOTE: As per Long Term Care Survey Guide, when life support systems are used, the facility must provide emergency electrical power with an emergency generator that is located on the premises.

Care plan must be completed.

MDS must be completed.

Potential tag: F241—Dignity

Potential tag: F272—Comprehensive Assessment

Potential tag: F279—Comprehensive Care Plan

Potential tag: F280—Comprehensive Care Plan Revision

Potential tag F281—Services are provided to Meet Professional Standard

Potential tag: F312—ADL Care for Dependent Residents

Potential tag: F327—Resident is Receiving Sufficient Fluid for Hydration

Potential tag F328—Treatment/Care for Special Needs

Potential tag: F385—Resident's Care Supervised by a Physician (must be on the monthly history and physical)

Potential tag: F441—Infection Control

Potential tag: F455—Emergency Electrical Power System

Potential tag: F456—Maintain Essential Equipment in Safe Condition

Potential tag: F498—Proficiency of Nursing Aides

GLUCOMETER

A glucometer is the device used to determine the concentration of glucose in the blood.

A blood sugar test must be done for all diabetic residents on a daily basis.

The machines must be tested for functionality on a daily basis to make sure that they are reading accurately. The test usually takes place during the 11-7 shift.

The results for "high" and "low" tests must always be documented.

NOTE: Failure to document the results of functionality tests of the glucometer may result in a citation!

Glucometer testing is done with the use of test strips and liquid which are usually supplied with the device. The reading should be within the manufacturer's acceptable range.

Taking The Resident's Blood Sugar Level:

The resident's fingertip MUST be cleaned before pricking the finger for blood.

NOTE: When doing finger-sticks for several residents, the glucometer MUST be cleaned with antimicrobial sanitary wipes in between tests.

NOTE: Failure to clean the glucometer between patient tests could result in a citation!

Nurses must wear gloves when doing finger-stick.

Nurses must change gloves and clean hands in between tests.

Finger-sticks must be done in privacy, not in the dining rooms, dayrooms or hallways.

NOTE: Failure to do finger-sticks in privacy can result in a citation!

Care plan must be completed.

MDS must reflect diagnosis.

Potential tag: F241—Dignity

Potential tag: F441—Infection Control

Potential tag: F456—Maintain Essential Equipment in Safe Condition

INFECTION AND ISOLATION

Infection control is very essential in health care. There is always an imminent risk for infection. Therefore facility must have an infection control program that prevents, investigates and controls infections.

Because of the multiple comorbidities and sharing of communal spaces, residents are at risk for infectious diseases. In an attempt to curb the spread of infectious diseases, facility must identify infected residents and move quickly to implement measures to prevent spread.

Facilities must have policies and procedures fulfilling the requirements of the Centers for Disease Control and Prevention to determine when residents should be placed on contact precautions or contact isolation. The following is a basic guide for infection control:

Must have doctor's order for contact precautions or contact isolation.

> Doctor must have clear, precise diagnosis for the isolation precautions and type of contact precaution/isolation needed.

> Contact precaution does not need a private room but contact isolation requires a private room.

> If a resident is showing signs and symptoms of a possible transmissible infection, e.g. frequent, loose and foul smelling bowel movements, it is advisable to put the resident on contact precautions until c-diff can be ruled out.

> Contact precautions must be written on the treatment administration record, medication administration record and the certified nursing assistant accountability record.

Dietary must be notified of all residents on isolation precautions so that disposable trays, dishes, and utensils can be utilized as necessary.

Must have sign on the resident's room door that says "STOP see nurse before entering."

Must have setup in hallway directly outside the room, with gowns, masks, and gloves (personal protective equipment).

Staff must be trained that under no circumstances should these personal protective equipment (PPE) be worn out of the room into the hallway and hands must be properly washed after removal.

For residents on isolation precautions for respiratory infections, it is advisable to ensure they have an adequate amount of tissue, hand sanitizer, and garbage pail in close proximity to the bed and teaching is provided and documented on sneezing, coughing, and blowing nose directly into a tissue.

Facility must have clear concise policy/procedure in place for handling garbage and linen from residents on isolation precautions in accordance with the Centers for Disease Control and Prevention regulations.

When a resident on isolation precautions is going to an outside appointment or being transferred to the hospital, this information must be shared with them.

Infection control is a mandatory ongoing in-service for all staff including but not limited to:

a. Proper hand hygiene
b. Proper usage of gloves
c. Proper cleaning of communal spaces such as handrails and equipment
d. Proper handling of linen

e. Proper food handling.

Residents with similar infections may cohort if they are on contact precautions, as determined by the facility's policy.

When the doctor gives an order to discontinue contact isolation, make sure it is discontinued in all areas.

It is important for the facility to recognize and contain infectious outbreaks. Three or more cases of the same type of infection over a limited space of time on the same unit should be monitored on a line listing.

Infection outbreaks in a facility are reportable to the Department of Health.

For all residents with any infections, it is important for the facility to have a monthly line listing of all these residents, which includes the following information:

a. Clearly differentiate between nosocomial or community-acquired infection
b. Type of infection
c. Site of infection
d. Date infection started
e. Type of antibiotic used
f. Start and end date of antibiotic use

At the end of the month, the completed list must be provided to the director of nursing/designee to tally the infection control stats for the facility and observe for patterns of clustered infections and any required in-service training.

Must be careful not to count prophylactic antibiotic therapy as a true infection when tallying up your monthly infections so as not to unnecessarily inflate your infection rate. Facility must adopt a protocol or criteria for diagnosing infections.

Some facilities have found it helpful to use nursing unit floor plan to identify infection clusters when analyzing infection patterns for expedient interventions.

NOTE: Surveyors at times will ask for the monthly line listing of infections on the units and will verify that residents with active infections are on this list.

The director of nursing, assistant director of nursing, infection control nurse and the medical director must familiarize themselves with the facility infection control practices, policies and procedures.

NOTE: Facilities must have alcohol based hand rub dispensers installed throughout the facility to promote infection control.

NOTE: The most prevalent sources of infection in any healthcare industry is wearing of gloves in communal spaces and poor hand hygiene!

Residents with the following conditions are at increased risk for infection:

1. Foley, Suprapubic or Urostomy catheters
2. Ostomies (tracheostomy, Gastrostomy, ileostomy, colostomy)
3. Intravascular catheters (dialysis catheters or other implanted ports)
4. Intravenous access (Heplock, PICC lines)
5. Wounds

MDS must reflect the diagnosis.

Care plan must be completed.

Potential tag: F272—Comprehensive Assessment

Potential tag: F274—Assessment after Significant Change

Potential tag: F279—Comprehensive Care Plan

Potential tag: F280—Comprehensive Care Plan Revision

Potential tag: F329—Unnecessary Drugs (resident is an on antibiotic to which the organism is resistive)

Potential tag: F371—Sanitary Conditions (plans to prevent infection through food handling)

Potential tag: F441—infection control, Prevent Spread, Clean Linen

Potential tag: F498—Proficiency of the Nurse Aides

IMMUNIZATION

Immunization of residents and staff is essential in preventing infections common to skilled nursing facilities. As part of the hiring process, new employees must have their tuberculosis screening done. All workers must be offered the flu shot if in flu season. To ensure proper record keeping, the following is best practice:

- Remind nurses to transcribe all immunization information on the immunization record in the medical records promptly as it is difficult to go back through months of completed medication administration records to retrieve this information.
- For facilities with electronic medication records, make sure information is entered in the immunization field also.
- When residents are transferred to the hospital, a copy of their immunization record must also be attached to the transfer record.
- Facilities must keep clear and concise records of all immunizations for residents and staff as this information is reportable yearly to the Department of Health in some states.
- Residents, family/legal representative and staff must be educated prior to immunization administration.
- Ensure care plan completion.
- MDS completion.

Influenza

It is the responsibility of the facility to ensure that residents and staff receive yearly *flu* shot. Accurate records must be kept for state review.

NOTE: Failure to keep accurate records may result in a citation!

1. Consent is required to administer the yearly *flu* shot to residents. Written or verbal consent must be obtained and may be clearly

written on the consent form. The form must be filed in the resident's active medical records.
2. If there is no representative and the resident is unable to give consent for the flu shot, this may be obtained at the discretion of the primary care doctor after careful review of the resident's medical history.
3. All staff must have proof of receiving the flu shot. It may be obtained in the facility or at the employee's private doctor's office. The facility must have a clear and precise record of who received it, who gave it, what date it was given and where it was given.

    1. For staff who received the flu shot, facility should have a system in place for identifying them such as issuing them a badge or sticker indicating that they received the flu shot.
    2. Facilities must have two separate typed lists department by department indicating all staff who received the flu shot and all staff who did not receive the flu shot.
    3. All staff who refused the flu shot are required to wear masks for a specific period in compliance with the Centers for Disease Control and Prevention (CDC) guidelines.

Tuberculosis (TB)

1. All new admissions to the facility must receive an initial PPD skin test for TB and have it repeated in ten to twenty-one days (based on facility policy) unless resident has a history of positive PPD test.
2. All residents and staff with history of positive PPD test must do chest x-ray at a maximum of every five years.
3. Readmitted residents do not require a repeat PPD test unless there is concern that the resident was exposed to tuberculosis while away from facility.
4. PPD testing is done annually. The order for the PPD test should have the month written alongside it so it is not missed.
5. A resident who had a negative PPD test that suddenly converts to positive result must have a full tuberculosis workup.
6. Consent is not required for PPD testing.

Pneumovax

Pneumovax is generally given every five years for residents over age fifty-five, but in an immunocompromised population, the schedule will vary at the discretion of the doctor. It is given to protect adults against certain strains of pneumonia.

1. All *pneumovax* must have a scheduled month and year next to them as part of the order so it is not missed.
2. Consent is required.

Potential tag: F272—Comprehensive Assessment

Potential tag: F280—Comprehensive Care Plan Revision

Potential tag: F334—influenza and pneumococcal immunization

Potential tag: F441—Infection Control

Potential tag: F501—Medical Director Involvement

CONSULTS

Consultation is sometimes necessary for diagnosis, treatment and management of certain medical conditions. Some consultants will generally see the residents in the facility but others require transportation of the resident to their office or another clinical setting.

When a consult is ordered, the resident must be seen within thirty days following the date of the order.

If the facility is unable to obtain an appointment within that window or an appointment is cancelled by the outside consultant, it is extremely important for the nurse to write a progress note to this effect and it is also prudent for the doctor to write a note that the consult is delayed but resident has no adverse effects. **NOTE: Failure to do this may result in a citation!**

It is very important for the consultant to receive a copy of all medications the resident is on to avoid overdosing or prescribing contraindicated medications.

When a resident is going to any outside appointment, it is prudent to send a copy of his or her advance directives so that in the event of an emergency, the Resident's/legal representative's wishes can be honored.

NOTE: When a resident returns from an appointment, the recommendations must be addressed with the doctor promptly and telephone orders obtained for any recommendation. This must be treated like any other acute situation.

Too often, these consults are left in the doctor's communication book, and this is considered delayed treatment, especially if there are recommendations for medication changes.

Many times consults have multiple recommendations. Nurses must read the recommendations carefully and ensure that all of them are addressed.

For in-house consultants there must be a clear and precise system that is clearly explained to all nurses and consultants.

NOTE: Too often residents go to outside appointments and return with the consultation form blank or just signed off. This is NOT sufficient! Results of ALL tests and consults must be obtained and addressed by the primary doctor!

NOTE: Podiatry consults are very essential especially for diabetics!

NOTE: Nursing staff must ensure that consultants such as dentists and podiatrists are changing gloves and washing hands between residents!

NOTE: Because a lot of consults require prior authorization from the insurance companies, it is important for this information to be obtained before resident goes out to appointment. Failure to do this, the consultant may not see the resident.

NOTE: Facility should have an assigned person who is responsible for obtaining all prior authorizations from insurance companies.

NOTE: For safety purposes, when a resident is going to an outside appointment, it is advisable for the facility to have a removable seatbelt that restraints the resident in the wheelchair and then ensure that the ambulette crew properly secures the resident's wheelchair in their vehicle.

Potential tag: F280—Comprehensive Care Plan Revision

Potential tag: F309—Provide Care/Services for Highest Well Being

Potential tag: F328--Treatment and Care for Special Care Needs

LABORATORY AND X-RAY SERVICES

Many illnesses and medications residents are receiving require frequent lab tests to monitor for development of other complications. Quality and timely lab services are essential to resident care. The following is best practice when labs are required:

1. All doctor's orders for labs should be documented on the 24 hour nursing report until the lab is completed, results are received, doctor is notified and doctor's recommendations are obtained.
2. Nursing documentation must be done in the resident's medical records indicating why the labs were ordered; when the labs were done; results received; doctor notification and doctor recommendations.
3. The doctor's recommendations such as holding or discontinuing medications and orders for repeat labs should also be carried on the 24 hour nursing report until labs are done and results again are received and doctor is notified.
4. When an order is given for a lab that requires several specimen collections, it is imperative that this be maintained on the 24 hour nursing report until ALL collections are obtained and results received. E.g. stool collection for c-difficle is sometimes ordered for three stool samples and upon chart review there is often only one or two collected!
5. When the nurse receives a doctor's order for bloodwork, the lab slips must be completed in entity, including the payer source and placed in the lab book so that when the lab technician arrives, there will be no delay in filling the paperwork.
6. Doctor's orders for stat labs must be transcribed promptly by the nurse and must be called to the lab.
7. Residents with conditions that limit blood draw to a particular arm must have that information displayed so that the lab technician is aware. E.g. residents with mastectomy or dialysis shunt.

8. If a resident refuses lab work or lab technician is unable to draw the blood due to poor venous access, this must be

   a. written on the lab sheet
   b. documented in the resident's medical record
   c. Doctor must be notified.

9. For residents with central lines if the facility policy allows for blood draw from these sites, the site should only be accessed by a facility nurse, not the outside lab technician.

10. Most lab results are received in 24 to 48 hours. If the lab return time is not efficient, this must be addressed promptly as it significantly impacts on residents' health.

11. If a resident is required to be without food (NPO) for a particular lab, this must be clearly reflected on the 24 hour nursing report, especially for the residents who are fed all night via tube feedings.

12. Many residents require routine labs weekly, monthly, every three or six months. The months that these labs are due should be written as part of the order. This will enable nurses reviewing doctor's monthly orders to be aware that these labs are due and therefore will fill the necessary paperwork and document on the 24 hour nursing report.

Radiological Studies:

The following are generally all done by the same diagnostic company:

   a. X-rays
   b. Sonograms
   c. Doppler Studies
   d. EKG
   e. Pacemaker checks

1. All doctor's orders for radiological studies should be documented on the 24 hour nursing report and in the resident's medical records until the test is completed, results received, doctor notification and doctor recommendations are obtained.

2. When a resident with a pacemaker is admitted, the diagnostic company should be notified so they can do routine pacemaker checks.
3. When scheduling radiological studies, verify if there are special instructions such as fasting, drinking extra fluids etc. and ensure that this is clearly documented on the 24 hour nursing report.
4. It is also extremely important to verify whether resident's medications need to be held
The doctor MUST give an order for holding the medication and for any special preparations required.
5. There are many other radiological services that are ordered by the doctor that must be done outside the facility e.g. CAT Scans; MRI, Studies of the GI tract etc. It is the responsibility of the facility to obtain authorization from the insurance company if necessary and arrange transportation for residents to get to these appointments.
6. Nursing MUST follow-up with ALL radiological, diagnostic and consultants to ensure completed results are obtained.

NOTE: Too often residents go to outside appointments and return with the consultation form blank or just signed off. This is NOT sufficient! Results of ALL tests and consults must be obtained!

Potential tag: F502—Provide and Obtain Lab Services-Quality/Timely

Potential tag: F503—Lab Services Provided by the Facility

Potential tag: F504—Lab Services only When Ordered by a Physician

Potential tag: F505—Physician promptly notified of lab results

Potential tag: F506—Facility Assist Resident in Transport to Lab (If done off premises)

Potential tag: F507—Lab Reports Filed in the Clinical Records

Potential tag: F508--Facility Provides and Obtains Radiological Services

Potential tag: F509—Radiological Services Meet Requirements

Potential tag: F510—Radiological/Diagnostic Studies Only When Ordered

Potential tag: F511—Radiological Studies—Promptly Notify Physician of Results

Potential tag: F512—Assist Resident with Transportation to Radiology

Potential tag: F513—Reports of X-rays and Diagnostic Services Filed in Resident's Records

DENTAL SERVICES

As per New York State regulations, all residents admitted to a skilled nursing facility must be seen by a dentist within 21 days. Residents must have a routine yearly dental consult done.

Conditions of the mouth, teeth and gums affect the Resident's ability to chew food and can result in several complications secondary to lack of adequate nutrition:

A. Weight lost
B. Development of pressure ulcers
C. Electrolyte imbalance.

For residents who utilize dentures, the following is best practice:

1. Certified nursing assistant accountability record must clearly reflect if resident have dentures and schedule for application and removal.
2. If dentures are lost or broken, urgent dental follow-up is needed.
3. Ensure dentures fit properly and report to nurse if too loose or resident with complaint of oral discomfort.
4. Ensure adequate mouth care is been provided at a minimum twice a day.
5. Remind staff to properly clean the mouths of residents who do not receive anything by mouth (NPO).
6. Remind nursing staff and dietary staff to always check trays and dishes for dentures at the end of meal times as confused residents often place them there.
7. When residents are transferred to the hospital, it is wise to document if they took their dentures with them (this applies to all other devices and personal property).

Potential tag: F411—Routine/Emergency Dental Services

HEARING AIDES AND GLASSES

Residents with assistive devices routinely require the services of a consultant to assess for deterioration or replacement of the devices. The following system of accountability is best practice:

1. Assistive devices must be documented on treatment administration record and certified nursing assistant accountability record.
2. Facility should have a system in place to ensure all assistive devices are permanently labelled.
3. The morning certified nursing assistant must retrieve <u>hearing aid</u> from the nurse, and the evening certified nursing assistant must return them to the nurse.
4. If the resident chooses to sleep with hearing aid or glasses the risks of lost and breakage must be clearly explained to the resident and it must be documented on the care plan.
5. If resident refuses to use, staff must sign "refuse" on the certified nursing assistant accountability record and care plan for same.
6. Ensure that resident is not refusing because device needs repairing.
7. Must have a schedule for battery replacement for hearing aids
8. Certified nursing assistants should notify nurse promptly if missing before signing "missing" on the accountability records.
9. Cannot sign "missing" for any prolonged period without indication of a follow-up consult with ENT, ophthalmology or audiology.
10. Frequency of which resident is seen by a consultant, where there are no issues, is predicated upon each facility's policy.
11. Glasses must be maintained in proper functioning order.
12. Residents with glasses should be seen at least once in a year by an ophthalmologist to assess for any visual changes.
13. Complete MDS.
14. Care plan must be completed.

NOTE: Any other prosthetic device such as dentures, artificial eye, artificial limb that is utilized by a resident must be clearly documented on the care plan and certified nursing assistant accountability record with clear instructions for application and removal. (The artificial eye MUST be on the treatment administration record as a task for the nurse!).

Potential tag: F272—Comprehensive Assessment

Potential tag: F279—Comprehensive Care Plan

Potential tag: F328—Treatment and Care for Special Care Needs

Potential tag: F313—Treatment/Devices to Maintain Hearing/Vision

CONSULTANT PHARMACIST

1. By State regulations, a consultant pharmacist must come in monthly to review the medications of all residents for discrepancies, such as the following:
   a. Incorrect orders, resulting in over or under-dosage
   b. Medication being given beyond the time it was ordered for
   c. Medications being given without a doctor's order
   d. Antibiotics and pain medications were started in a timely manner
   e. Consults and labs required with medication usage not being done
   f. Medications usage with the wrong diagnosis
   g. Use of multiple medications that have the same effect
   h. Potential for adverse interactions between medications
   i. PRN medications that have not being used for over 30 days (e.g., Tylenol)
   j. Use of prn medication and effectiveness is written on the pain scale and the site of pain is documented on the back of medication administration record or the electronic medication record administration.
   k. Assess for psychiatrist's attempt at gradual dose reduction
   l. Medication storage must be locked with narcotics double locked
   m. Emergency box with no expired medications
   n. All opened vials have open and discard dates
   o. System in place for receipt, storage, dispense, documentation and disposition of controlled drugs.
   p. Ensuring nurses are signing the medication and treatment records
   q. Vital signs parameters required with certain medications are been done
   r. Orders that require special instructions have those written as part of the order e.g. two nurses to be present and sign for removal and discard of Duragesic patch

  s. Medications not recommended for use in elderly population are been administered

  t. Are there significant recent changes to a resident as a result of a medication

  u. Refrigerated medications stored at the right temperature

2. These consultants either sign on the current monthly order sheets or often have their own form at the back of the nursing notes that they sign on.

3. When their recommendations are given to nursing management, it is advisable to make a copy for your records so you know what is distributed to the nurses and the doctors when you need to retrieve them.

4. All recommendations must have a clearly written response as to how the problem was corrected in the box next to the identified problem.

5. If the doctor does not agree with the recommendation, just like with all consults, he must document on the form why he disagrees.

6. **NOTE:** Surveyors generally ask for at least the last six months of these documents and can go further back if they encounter any discrepancies in the medications.

Potential tag: F329—Drug Regimen is free from Unnecessary Drugs

Potential tag: F332—Free of Medication Error Rates of 5% or more

Potential tag F333—Residents are Free of Significant Medication Errors

Potential tag: F385—Resident's Care Supervised by a Physician

Potential tag F425—Facility Provides Drugs and Biologicals

Potential tag: F428—Drug Regimen Reviewed Monthly

Potential tag F431—Proper Labelling/Storage of Drugs and Biologicals

REHABILITATION SERVICES

The primary goal of rehabilitation services is restoration of some or all of physical and mental functions lost as a result of illness or injury. Rehabilitation also includes assisting residents to compensate for deficits that cannot be reversed. Therapy serves to help individuals restore the use of muscles and bones, regain the ability to do normal daily tasks, correct speech disorders.

Many residents require assistive devices such as splints, braces etc. to support weakened extremities, reduce pain and prevent contracture.

In an effort to ensure qualitative care, the rehab department and nursing department must work collaboratively together to ensure that all recommendations from rehabilitation to nursing as well as the nursing department to the rehabilitation department are clearly documented and adhered to by both departments. The following is best practice for communication between these departments:

1. A doctor's order is required for the initiation of any rehabilitation services.
2. Rehabilitation department must assess all new admissions, re-admissions, Residents with significant changes, residents with cognitive or functional decline and residents that had accidents/incidents for the need for rehabilitative services.
3. **NOTE:** Any referrals from the nursing department to the rehabilitation department require a nursing progress note clearly delineating the areas of decline and why rehabilitation services are needed. A nursing to rehabilitation communication form must also be completed and provided to rehabilitation department.
4. All recommendations from the rehabilitation department to the nursing department must be clearly documented on the certified nursing assistant accountability record and the resident's care plan. These include splints, devices, wheelchairs, cushions, floor

ambulation, range of motion, start and end of therapy, change in ADL functions, and eating utensils. A doctor's order for these is recommended.

5. It is advisable to have a clear *rehab-to-nursing* communication form.

6. The rehabilitation department should NOT flag their recommendations in the chart as nurses often ignore them or file them away without following through on the recommendations.

7. It is recommended that a staff member of the rehabilitation department follows up on all recommendations with the nursing department to ensure accountability, implementation and compliance.

8. It is recommended that rehabilitation department takes all documentation to a central nursing person (s) for signature. The rehabilitation staff member can also take all their correspondence to morning meetings, as all nurse managers do attend and all paperwork can be signed and promptly returned to the rehabilitation department.

9. The Director of Nursing and the rehab head should determine a central person who will receive a copy of all these rehab communications and ensure that they are appropriately transcribed on the certified nursing assistant accountability record and the care plan.

10. Rehab department should put in front of resident's accountability record a picture of all devices and splint and instructions on how to apply them.

11. Rehab department should have signed in-services that the nursing staff was trained on how to apply a device.

12. **NOTE**: Residents that require assistive devices at mealtimes such as built up spoon or scoop dish involve the coordination of the dietary department and the occupational therapy unit of the rehabilitation department.

13. **NOTE:** It is advisable for all unit managers to get a weekly list of all devices, splints, cushions, range of motion and ambulation programs. Etc. from the rehabilitation department. Nursing supervisors must ensure that these are properly documented on the care plan and on the certified nursing assistant accountability record.

14. During daily rounds, nurses must ensure all devices are properly applied per resident's individual schedule.
15. Any resident that is started on rehabilitation must have a doctor's order to initiate the rehabilitation services.
16. Surveyors will generally check for the following:

   a. A doctor's order for rehab services carried on the monthly doctor's orders
   b. A physical or occupational therapy assessment
   c. Rehab recommendation transcribed on the certified nursing assistant accountability record and care plan
   d. Implementation of the recommended device
   e. Proper application of the devices per individual schedules
   f. The schedule for applying and removing the device or devices,
   g. Protocol for checking for positive and negative effects of the device (pressure, ulceration etc.)
   h. Schedule in place for cleansing device
   i. Alternatives when device is removed for washing
   j. Supervision of nursing assistants during floor ambulation programs to ensure compliance with rehabilitation recommendations.
   k. Evaluation of residents receiving range of motion for signs of improvement or otherwise.
   l. Observe to see if range of motion exercises are provided per the plan of care
   m. Does MDS reflect required device or rehabilitation service.
   n. Proof of a care plan and its implementation.

Potential tag: F311—Treatment/Services to Improve/Maintain ADLs

Potential tag: F317—No Reduction in ROM Unless Unavoidable

Potential tag: F318—Increase/Prevent Decrease in Range of Motion

Potential tag: F385—Resident's Care Supervised by a Physician (must be on monthly orders)

Potential tag: F406—Provide/Obtain Specialized Rehab Services

Potential tag: F407—Rehab Services Had a Physician Order/Services Provided by a Qualified Person

CHANGES IN ACTIVITIES OF DAILY LIVING

Many residents admitted to skilled care facilities are placed for long term care due to inability to meet their own activities of daily living (ADL) and/or the unavailability of someone to care for them in the community. Because of physical limitations or cognitive impairments, many of these residents require assistance with their activities of daily living.

As per The Long Term Care Manual, the goals for these residents are:

a). Resident that enter the facility without any limitation to their range of motion must not experience reduction in their range of motion unless the resident's clinical condition demonstrates that a reduction is unavoidable.

b). Residents that are admitted with limitations to range of motion get the treatment and services needed to increase their range of motion or prevent further decrease.

Any decline in a resident's activities of daily living must be assessed and be determined as either avoidable or non-avoidable.

Activities of daily living include the Resident's ability or inability to self-perform the following activities:

a). Eat
b). Transfer
c). Toilet
d). Ambulate
e). Bathe
f). Dress and
g). Groom

Ongoing review of a resident's ability to maintain current level of ADL must be done to prevent undetected decline.

Nurses must always encourage the certified nursing assistants to report any changes they observe to resident's level of care as they are more likely to be the first set of caregivers to detect ADL declines.

NOTE: The survey team does look at a sample of residents' activities of daily living (ADL) and compare to previous numbers to see if there has been a change. If there is a decline, the contributory factors must be clearly documented (e.g., decrease in mobility secondary to comorbidities, worsening of illness, or worsening dementia).

Residents with changes in two or more areas of their ADLs must be referred to MDS coordinator for evaluation for significant change and to rehab department to evaluate for need for rehabilitative services.

Care plan, MDS and certified nursing assistant accountability record must accurately reflect the level of care resident requires. **NOTE:** Failure to do this may generate a citation in the area of proper documentation!

Surveyors are likely to observe resident receiving care and compare to the written plan of care to ensure resident is receiving the level of care documented.

NOTE: The certified nursing assistants often wrongly change the level of care resident requires on the certified nursing assistant accountability record and fail to notify the nurse. They may also fail to communicate their observations with the nurse so that the records can be adjusted after properly assessing the resident.

Potential tag: F272—Comprehensive Assessment

Potential tag: F279—Comprehensive Care Plan

Potential tag: F280—Comprehensive Care Plan Revision

Potential tag: F310—ADLs Do Not Decline Unless Unavoidable

Potential tag: F311—Treatment/Services to Improve/Maintain ADLs

Potential tag: F312—ADL Care Provided for Dependent Residents

ENVIRONMENTAL ROUNDS

The environment in a facility is very important to the overall care of the residents. The environment impacts on infection control, risk for accidents/incidents, weight management and quality of life. Nurses should make rounds on units at the start of their shift. However, the facility should have an interdisciplinary team comprising of the Administrator, the Director of Housekeeping, the Director of Maintenance and the nursing management for the purpose of making weekly rounds on the environment and to observe for the following:

Dining Room

1. During mealtime, see aforementioned on meal observation.
2. Ensure suction machine is functional.
3. Suction machine is covered during non-mealtimes.
4. Tables and environment properly cleaned after meals.
5. Normal saline solution on the suction machine has not expired.
6. The suction machine cord can extend the entire length (width) of the dining room.
7. A clean homelike environment is maintained.
8. All medication and treatment carts are locked and nurses are assisting at mealtimes.
9. The area is well lit, clean, in appropriate temperature and free of odor
10. Residents are not too tightly seated or packed

Hallways

1. All objects in the hallway are lined to one side.
2. All exits and entrances to residents' rooms are not blocked
3. Ensure that hallways are well lite and clean
4. The State and Ombudsman's phone numbers are highly visible.
5. The current recreational calendar is posted in a highly visible area at residents' eye level.

6. The current menu is also posted in highly visible areas at residents' eye level.
7. No visible spills anywhere
8. Handrails are not loose.
9. Residents been transported to/from showers are properly covered.
10. Residents are clean and well groomed
11. Residents' fingernails are cut
12. Staff respect resident's privacy and dignity by knocking on doors.
13. No odors
14. No broken equipment are observed on the floor

Medication Cart

1. Cart must are clean with no expired medications stocked.
2. All open bottles are properly and legibly dated.
3. Ointments and inhalers must be individually bagged or boxed and are properly labeled.
4. Narcotics are in locked bin.
5. Carts are locked.

Treatment Cart

1. Each resident must have their own creams and/or ointments; these cannot be shared between residents.
2. All saline solutions and other open solutions are legibly dated.
3. Dressings are in sufficient supply.
4. Carts are locked.

Nursing Station

1. No food in open view in the nursing station
2. Medical records are not easily viewable by other residents and visitors.
3. No hanging lists with residents' names and/or room numbers are easily visible by visitors or residents
4. The call bell system is functioning

Residents' Rooms

1. Residents' rooms are clean and in homelike appearance
2. The call bell is working
3. No extra linen is put in each room because this may generate an infection control citation as it is under the presumption that the extra linen will be taken to other residents' rooms
4. The space between objects placed on top of closet and the ceiling is not less than 18 inches
5. There are no odors in the rooms
6. There are no risks for accidents/incidents (e.g., bed too high, resident positioned close to the edge, jagged-edged furniture)
7. Urinals are clearly labeled when there are two male room-mates
8. No urinals are placed on over bed tables when meals are on the table
9. Rooms in appropriate temperature 71-81 degrees
10. Water is running in appropriate temperature—not too hot or too cold
11. The room is not excessively cluttered. Care plan is in place for non-compliant residents
12. All IV, GT, oxygen, and nebulizer tubing are legibly dated.
13. Food storage at bedside is in a sealable container, legibly labeled and dated
14. Ensure alarms are working and floor mats are in place or properly put away
15. Make sure beds are neatly made and the linen is clean
16. Ensure adequate lighting
17. If there is a water pitcher at bedside, make sure it is dated
18. Privacy curtains in place and functioning
19. All electrical devices in use have records of inspection by maintenance department
20. If the resident is in bed are comfortably positioned in bed

Maintenance Department Environmental Rounds:

The general maintenance and upkeep of the facility's appearance is the primary responsibility of the Environmental Unit. The unit must ensure that:

1. Water is running at acceptable temperature in the range of 95-120 degrees
2. Air temperature is in the range of 71-81 degrees
3. Maintenance logs are checked and are signed off daily
4. Pest control logs are checked daily and are followed up with the contractor as needed
5. There is an adequate amount of emergency water supply
6. Handrails in corridors and elevators are properly secured
7. No torn armrests on wheelchairs
8. Broken equipment are removed from the environment
9. No loose wires
10. There is adequate functioning of the ventilation system including smoking room
11. No doors have door stops to jar them open!
12. General maintenance and upkeep of facility's appearance
13. Sprinkler heads are clean and not blocked
14. Exits are clearly marked and not blocked
15. Maintain a log of maintenance all residents' personal electrical equipment e.g. coffeemakers etc.

Potential tag: F240—Care and Environment Promote Quality of Life

Potential tag F241—Dignity and Respect of Individuality

Potential tag: F252 Safe, Clean, Comfortable, Homelike Environment

Potential tag F254—Clean Bed and Linen

Potential tag: F256—Adequate and Comfortable Lightening

Potential tag: F456—Essential Equipment in Safe Condition

Potential tag: F460—Bedroom Assure Full Visual Privacy

Potential tag F463—Residents call bell systems in Rooms/Toilets

Potential tag: F464—Requirements for Space for Activities and Dining

Potential tag: F465—Environment is Safe, Functional, Sanitary and Comfortable

Potential tag: F466—Emergency Water Available

Potential tag: F467—Adequate outside Ventilation

Potential tag: F468—Corridors have firmly secured handrails

Potential tag: F469—Maintain Effective Pest Control Program

WATER AND ROOM TEMPERATURES

As part of maintaining a safe and homelike environment, particular attention must be paid to room temperature levels and water temperature. The elderly are very susceptible to loss of body heat through the skin secondary to decrease in fat and muscles under the skin. Many medical conditions can also result in hands and feet feeling constantly cold e.g. low blood pressure and circulatory problems. The elderly are at increased risks for burns secondary to thinning of the skin.

> The facility's maintenance director must have a system in place for ensuring that water temperature is checked and logged daily.

> The water is not the exact same temperature every time tested; therefore, the log must reflect the variations observed.

> **NOTE:** The acceptable water temperature should be in the range of 90 to 120 degrees.

> Staff should be trained to report if water temperature is too hot or too cold.

> Aside from the maintenance director, *all* staff must be trained or in-serviced on what the appropriate room temperature is for residents' rooms and be reminded to check same every time they enter residents' rooms.

> **NOTE:** The acceptable room temperature should always be in the range of 71 to 81 degrees.

> **NOTE:** It is advisable to dress the elderly residents in layers to ensure their comfort.

Potential tag: F257—Comfortable and Safe Temperature Levels

NOISE LEVELS

In an ongoing attempt to ensure a home-like environment, noise levels are very important. Facility must be mindful of how difficult it is for residents to concentrate or maintain homeostasis when there is excessive noise in the background.

If a facility is undergoing construction, it is advisable to inform residents and the families/legal representatives prior to initiation and scheduled work hours and document same.

Staff members must be trained to minimize yelling, loud talking or loud music playing (unless for recreational programs) on the units.

Every attempt should be made to operate noisy equipment such as vacuums and buffers during the day time.

NOTE: Facility should pay particular attention to residents' complaints of staff talking loudly on the units during the evening and the night shifts.

Alarms and call bells should be answered timely to minimize noise!

Potential tag: F258—Maintenance of Comfortable Sound Levels.

FOOD STORAGE, PREPARATION
AND DISTRIBUTION

Food complaints are often the number one complaints in facilities!

Foods must be handled and stored in a proper manner to prevent outbreaks of food borne illnesses. Food borne illnesses are often manifested by nausea, vomiting and diarrhea which can lead to dehydration and subsequently death for immunocompromised residents!

Food must be properly handled from the time of receipt from the vendor to the time of consumption. The following is a basic guide for proper food management:

Storage:

1. Boxes of delivered foods should NEVER be stored on the floor. Facility must have arrangement with vendor as to where food will be placed in the event it is delivered during off duty hours.
2. Staff should ensure that food received from vendors is checked for proper packaging, received at the right temperature and not damage or spoiled.
3. Stored items should NOT be obstructing the sprinklers
4. Foods must be stored at the recommended temperature. Kitchen must maintain a log to show refrigerator temperatures are checked daily and in the correct range.
5. Foods that require dry storage must be properly secured. Often the kitchen is in the basement and facility must be very mindful of even the slightest leaks or storage location close to water source.
6. Food storage and preparation areas should be pest free! Food Service Director/Maintenance must maintain a log of frequency of visits from the pest control contractor.

7. Kitchens are often in the basement or on the lower level; therefore, it is very important to keep food clear of sewers and waste disposal pipes and to ensure proper working ventilation.
8. Dry and refrigerated stored food items must be clearly labelled as to when they are to be discarded.
9. Foods in walk in closets or refrigerators MUST be stored OFF the floor.
10. When storing foods, be mindful of juices from raw foods such as meats dripping on other foods!
11. Canned goods should not be dented or punctured.
12. Meats and other food items should not be thawed sitting out on counters!
13. The time for cooling cooked foods should NOT exceed six hours.
14. Expired food must not be served.

Kitchen Staff:

15. All dietary staff must wear hair protectors.
16. Staff must be trained to wash hands frequently with soap and water.
17. Foods should not be handled with bare hands. Gloves, tongs, spatulas etc. should be used accordingly.
18. Hand jewelry and other dangling jewelry is not recommended for dietary staff while on duty.
19. Gloves MUST be changed between tasks to prevent cross contamination.
20. Staff with any infectious or communicable diseases or skin lesions should be excluded from food preparation.

Environment:

21. No dirt, grime, food or grease must be allowed to build up on utensils, floors, walls, ceilings, fans, ventilation systems or sprinkler systems.
22. Meat slices must be properly cleaned and covered.
23. Clean sanitized cutting boards between uses.

24. Ensure proper cleaning of frequently used items such as knives, can openers, blenders, slicers between uses.
25. When chopping meats etc. and dealing with chemicals staff must be mindful of flying parts that can land in other foods or clean areas causing contamination.

Food Preparation:

26. Foods MUST always be prepared at the right temperature.
27. Food preparers should have a list of required temperatures for individual food preparation and reheating guidelines readily available and are frequently in-serviced on these.
28. Kitchen workers must be frequently in-serviced on these.

Food Distribution to Residents:

29. Food Service Director must ensure that food temperatures are maintained at correct temperature while on tray lines, steam tables, food trucks, arrival on individual units to the point of serving to the residents AT ALL TIMES!
30. Hot foods must be served hot and cold foods must be served cold! (Eating food when hot prevent bacteria consumption).

Washing and Sanitizing of Dishes:

31. Facility dishwasher must be operating according to the manufacturer's specifications for washing, rinsing and sanitizing of dishes.
32. The washing temperature of dishwashing machines should be in the range of 120 to 165 degrees.
33. The rinsing temperature of the dishwashing machine should be in the range of 160 to 180 degrees.
34. For manual washing of dishes

    a. Scrape food off of dishes
    b. Wash using hot water and recommended detergent
    c. Rinsing with hot water

    d. Sanitizing by immersing in hot water or a recommended chemical solution. (Food Service Director should have clear guidelines on these products!).

    e. Allow to air dry.

35. Facility should ensure it employs adequate amount of staff in the kitchen to ensure compliance with the regulatory requirements.

Potential tag: F362—Sufficient Dietary Support Personnel

Potential tag: F371—Sanitary food Procurement, Preparation, Distribution and Storage

Potential tag: F441—Infection Control

Potential tag: F456—Essential Equipment in Safe Operating Condition

Potential tag: F465—Environment is Safe, Functional, Sanitary and Comfortable

Potential tag: F469—Maintain Effective Pest Control Program

GARBAGE DISPOSAL

As part of ensuring a safe, clean, sanitary and homelike environment, surveyors will inspect the way the facility handles storage and disposes of garbage.

1. The Housekeeping Director must ensure that the environment is free of soiled linen and garbage buildup, especially on off hours when there is limited staffing.
2. Garbage and soiled linen storage areas inside the facility must be locked and secured with adequate ventilation to minimize odors.
3. **NOTE:** Staff must be in-serviced to ensure all garbage and soiled linen are properly tied in plastic bags before leaving residents' rooms to minimize odor.
4. Outside garbage containers must be properly covered with no leaks.
5. Garbage receptacles MUST be properly covered when transporting them to the dumpster
6. Outside garbage area should be maintained in a sanitary condition to prevent attracting pests.

Potential tag: F372—Proper Disposal of Garbage and Refuse.

DISASTER PROTOCOL

Residents and families/legal representative must have a sense of security that in the event of a facility wide emergency such as fire or severe weather, there is a protocol in place for their safe removal and contingency plans for appropriate temporary placement.

Fire and Safety teaching is mandatory for all staff members and there should be schedules in place for drills to ensure appropriate response.

The facility must have emergency or disaster protocol in place.

A disaster drill must be conducted at a minimum of twice a year with signed in-services and a clear outline of the nature of the drill.

Staff must be able to clearly understand the facility's plan in the event of a disaster.

Fire drills must be conducted on each shift at a minimum every three months and signed in-services logs must be maintained.

Fire safety is an ongoing mandatory in-service for all staff members.

Facility must have agreements with other facilities to transfer residents in the event of an emergency.

An elopement drill is considered a disaster drill and should be done and documented yearly!

Surveyors will often ask staff about the facility's disaster protocol:

a. What do you do when the fire alarm goes off?

b. What is the fire acronym for the facility? E.g. ARCE-Alarm, rescue, contain, extinguish

c. What are the codes use in the facility in the event of an emergency?

d. E.g. Dr. Red for fire; Code blue for medical Emergency; Code Black for missing resident etc.

e. Where are fire extinguishers located and the types of extinguishers?

f. How do you use a fire extinguisher?

g. What is the response when a smoke or a fire is located in a resident's room?

h. What is the protocol when a resident is missing?

NOTE: Staff in facilities in areas prone to hurricanes, tornadoes, floods, earthquakes should be trained how to respond to these.

Potential tag: F517—Written Plans to Meet Emergencies/Disaster

Potential tag: F518—Train all Staff; Emergency Procedures/Drills.

QUALITY ASSESSMENT AND ASSURANCE
(OR QUALITY IMPROVEMENT)

Quality assessment and assurance incorporates every aspect of care and activities in the facility. It should be a daily interdisciplinary routine to assess for issues which impede quality care, issues with inherent potential for harm either physically and mentally or issues that violate residents' rights.

The purpose for the quality assessment and assurance committee is for the facility to identify internal deficiencies and develop and implement plans to correct them.

The quality assessment and assurance meetings should be attended by all department heads for the purpose of coming up with plans of correction for any areas of deficiencies in their departments.

It is advisable to have RN unit managers, some LPNS and certified nursing assistants attend these meetings.

All previously identified survey deficiencies and the plans of correction should be an ongoing part of quality assurance.

Facility must have a quality assessment and assurance committee that meets at a minimum of every three months.

Quarterly topics must be relevant and focused on improving quality of care.

NOTE: Good practice is for nursing management and the administrator to generate the list of pertinent topics and discuss and distribute to the department heads to ensure all areas with inherent potential for deficient practice are addressed.

All staff must be able to identify members of the quality assurance committee in the event they have issues and concerns they will know who to address them with.

NOTE: The facility must have ongoing QA projects that all staff members are trained or in-serviced on.

NOTE: Surveyors generally pick staff at random and ask them about the facility's ongoing QA projects, so aside from in-services, it is advisable to post the contents of these projects in highly visualized areas.

The head of the QA committee must be ready to discuss with surveyors the ongoing QA projects for the facility.

Some good ongoing QA topics are:

a. Accident/incident prevention—Resident safety
b. Fall prevention
c. Customer service
d. Abuse prevention
e. Respecting resident's privacy-knocking on doors
f. All staff answering call bells
g. Maintaining residents' privacy or HIPAA
h. Pressure ulcer prevention
i. The five star quality measures

Potential tag: F520—QAA Committee Members Meet Quarterly

MORNING INTERDISCIPLINARY MEETINGS

Morning interdisciplinary meetings provide daily quality assessment and assurance for the facility. It sets the tone and direction for the day.

Is it really necessary to read the twenty-four-hour nursing report verbatim for *all* department heads?

When all department heads are in the morning meeting, the following information must be reported clearly:

a. All admissions must be mentioned
b. All discharges
c. Pending discharges
d. All accidents and incidents
e. Any new skin breaks
f. Any elopements and/or attempts
g. Any issues (e.g., broken beds, unclean rooms, wrong diet, room and water temperature issues)
h. Any off shift room changes

Department heads' responsibilities after morning meeting aside from their regular duties:

Social services:

Ensure that nurses gave all discharged residents the discharge/transfer paperwork. All residents were given their bill of rights upon admission. Families were contacted for accidents/incidents, skin breaks, elopements or room changes. Follow-up on complaints or grievances discussed at morning meeting.

Maintenance:

Make sure that any equipment involved in accidents/incidents are quickly assessed/fixed and that a report is given to the director of nursing/designee and that any water or room temperature issues are promptly addressed. Should also check all maintenance logs at each nursing station.

Housekeeping:

Ensure that the rooms of permanently discharged residents are stripped and cleaned and ready for the next admission. Safely secure the belongings of discharged residents; Search for missing clothing and laundry complaints.

Assistant administrator (or designee):

Ensure that rental equipment for hospitalized/discharged residents are secured and returned to vendors.

Rehabilitation:

Evaluates residents with accidents/incidents and skin breaks for any device changes or to be picked up for therapy and assess all admissions/re-admissions.

Admissions:

Ensure that all residents who were discharged or transferred were properly discharged from the system to prevent error in documentation and billing.

After department heads depart from the meeting, a nursing meeting should follow where they spend time doing chart review and medication reconciliation for all admissions and re-admissions.

Nursing should ensure all episodic care plans are updated also, and that new ones initiated.

JANE GABBIDON

Whether or not the report is read in the morning meeting, it is prudent for the Director of Nursing/Designee to go through the entire report. You will be amazed how many little, subtle things you pick up that the nurse skipped over when reading the report.

Best practice is that after reading the report, the Director of Nursing and the Assistant Director of Nursing should divide the 24 hour nursing report and review the documentation of all residents on the report. Again you will be amazed at the discrepancies between the reports and the charts. Call staff to come in and write late entry or clarification notes. Once they know that you are reviewing the notes daily and there is a possibility they will be called in, you will be amazed how quickly the quality of the documentation improves. This also quickly corrects any discrepancies and encourages proper documentation. **NOTE: This is a good method for preventing poor quality of care and avoidable citations!**

Electronic Medical Records Morning Meetings

It is advisable for the Director of Nursing and the Assistant Director of Nursing to read the progress notes for *all disciplines* for the past twenty-four hours prior to morning meeting and have a list of all of the aforementioned pertinent information.

1. After department heads depart, all disciplines progress notes written the previous day should be reviewed by the nursing team and each nurse should update acute changes in the relevant care plans.
2. Documentation from the other disciplines that require nursing follow-up should be done and nurses should inform doctors of issues that require follow-up.
3. As part of the medication reconciliation for new admissions or re-admissions, the doctor's orders and the certified nursing assistant accountability records should be reviewed.
4. It is also advisable for the nursing team to review all of the doctors' orders written the previous day for any discrepancies to prevent avoidable medication errors.

MAINTENANCE OF RESIDENT'S CLINICAL RECORDS

The facility must maintain clinical records on each resident that are complete, accurate, readily accessible and organized.

The clinical record must contain

1. Sufficient information to clearly identify the resident
2. A record of all resident assessments
3. The plan of care and services provided
4. The results of any pre-admission screening (PRI, Screen, PSARR)
5. Progress notes

Documentation should show a clear picture of the resident's status prior to admission, status upon admission and services provided while in the facility with any response to treatment or change in condition.

Documentation should be ongoing and interdisciplinary and any change to the resident or the resident's condition must be documented.

NOTE: If care and services provided are not documented, then there is NO way of proving that same was done!

A facility may not release information that is resident identifiable to the public.

NOTE: The facility is responsible for safeguarding resident's records against lost, destruction or unauthorized use.

NOTE: When a resident is discharged, the facility is responsible for having the records accessible for a minimum of seven years.

NOTE: With the rapid evolving changes to social media, staff must be mindful **NOT** to discuss or post any information about a resident or incident within the facility on any public websites!

Potential tag: F514—Resident's Records Must be Complete, Accurate and Accessible

Potential tag: F515—Retention of Resident's Clinical Records

Potential tag: F516—Facility Must Safeguard Resident's Clinical Records and Cannot

Release Resident's information to the public.

ROSTER MATRIX, CASPER REPORTS
OR QUALITY INDICATOR REPORT

It is best practice to pull the facility's CASPER report and Roster Matrix at least monthly and check for the areas that residents are triggering for on submitted MDS and ensure these areas have adequate care plans in place. This is also a good tool for knowing if information submitted on the MDS is accurate. This is also another step in quality assessment and assurance.

FIVE STAR RATING

Five star rating is now the newest way the public evaluates skilled care facilities!

Five-star rating was implemented by Centers for Medicare and Medicaid Services (CMS) to rate facilities. Areas that they review are the following:

a. Survey
b. Quality measures
c. Staffing

There are eleven identified quality measures:

1. pressure ulcers
2. pain
3. ADL decline
4. catheters
5. falls with injury
6. high-risk pressure ulcers
7. pain adjusted
8. physical restraints
9. UTI;
10. long-term residents' (over one hundred days) usage of antipsychotic medications;
11. short term residents' usage of antipsychotic medication.

These quality measures are gleamed from submitted MDS forms for our residents, hence the importance of ensuring the accuracy of information submitted.

It is highly recommended that facilities look at these quality measures and have ongoing quality assurance programs for improvement.

In an effort to remain competitive, of course, a facility's five-star rating is important. Many hospitals use the five-star ratings to predict how well a nursing home does in preventing re-hospitalizations. There are facilities with less stars that provide quality service and that is why it is so crucial for a facility to clearly communicate to hospitals all the services it can provide so that re-hospitalizations are minimized.

Ongoing quality assurance and assessment in these areas has a twofold purpose

1. Residents will receive care that will promote maintenance or enhancement of their quality of life.
2. It will make hospitals and families feel comfortable in referring admissions to the facility. **NOTE:** This enhances the image of the facility positively!

RE-HOSPITALIZATION

Re-hospitalization rates is also one of the newest ways nursing homes are being evaluated by the public!!

As long-term care providers, we are aware that aside from the excellent care provided by hospitals, there are some negative outcomes predicated upon excessive hospitalizations of elderly residents. Frequent removal of residents from their homelike environment has the potential for increased confusion, weight loss, and skin breakdown.

NOTE: In an attempt to reduce excessive nursing-home-to-hospital traffic, there are now monetary fines against the discharging hospitals when residents are readmitted before thirty days. Eventually, these monetary charges will also apply to the nursing home!

Excessive re-hospitalization under thirty days may reflect poorly on the quality of care provided by the nursing home, which subsequently can impact on the relationship between the skilled nursing facility and the hospital. If a resident is discharged from the nursing home to the community and is readmitted to the hospital all under thirty days, this counts as re-hospitalization. In an attempt to minimize excessive hospitalization, the following are considered best practices:

1. A warm hand off from hospital nurse to nursing home nurse would be helpful.
2. Upon review of a resident's medications and medical history prior to and during admission, the INTERACT Quality Improvement Tool is a good guide for addressing and actively treating acute or potentially acute conditions from the admission shift.
3. MD should determine root cause for any acute symptoms and move to treat them quickly as some conditions lead to very rapid deterioration. (E.g., a resident admitted with loose BM and, as per hospital records, *C. difficile* toxin assay results pending.

If the loose BM is left untreated within twenty-four hours, resident may become dehydrated and have poor oral intake, increased confusion, and abnormal vital signs.

4. The INTERACT Stop and Watch Tool is also another great asset. *All* staff should be trained, in-serviced and encouraged to utilize this tool to alert the nurse when there are changes in the resident's condition. A housekeeper is sometimes at the resident's bedside more frequently than the nurse, and that is why it is important for all staff to be trained.

5. It is a good practice to keep all new admissions and readmissions on twenty-four-hour nursing report for thirty days. The first seven days could be detailed documentation, and day eight to thirty just their vital signs, but at least resident will be monitored by a nurse or aide every shift.

6. A facility should know its readmission rate and the diagnoses for readmissions.

7. Ensure the facility has a follow-up post-discharge plan to the community.

8. Facility should have a skilled checklist of the services it can provide, including but not limited to IV hydration, IV antibiotics, EKG monitoring, bladder scan, etc., and share with the hospitals.

9. There are programs such as PointRight that have excellent tools to track and reduce re-hospitalization rates in long-term care facilities.

10. Medication reconciliation with twenty-four hours of admission is crucial.

NOTE: The management must NOT compromise the health of residents because of possible penalty arising from re-hospitalization within 30 days!

PAYMENT

Most residents in nursing homes payer source is Medicare or Medicaid. Facilities are required to submit Minimum Data Set (MDS) assessments on residents as previously mentioned. The level of care a resident requires generates what is called a RUG score (Resource Utilization Group). Medicare and Medicaid RUGS are different. For the purpose of this discussion, the following is only an outline to explain the lettering of RUG scores.

MEDICARE RUG CATEGORIES

The following is a Medicare RUG outline to provide a basic understanding of the lettering and how RUG scores are obtained.

R	Rehabilitation
U	Ultrahigh (720 rehab mins per week).
V	Very high (500 rehab mins per week).
H	High (300 rehab mins per week).
M	Medium (150 rehab mins per week).
X	Extensive services attached to a rehab score. *X* is higher ADL score (e.g., RUX).
L	Extensive services attached to a rehab score. *L* is for lower ADL score (e.g., RUL).
ES	Extensive services.
H	Special care high.
L	Special care low.
C	Clinically complex.
B	Behaviors.
P	Reduced physical function.

E D C B A	These letters reflect the total ADL score, with *E* being the highest (resident is more dependent) and *A* being the lowest (resident is less dependent).
Number 2	Under special care high, special care low, clinically complex, behaviors, and reduced physical, number 2 means resident has signs/symptoms of depression.

Number 1	Under special care high, special care low, clinically complex, behaviors, and reduced physical, number 1 means resident has *no* signs/symptoms of depression.
ES3, ES2 ES1 (Extensive care RUGS)	Under Extensive services, the numbers 3, 2, and 1 are different. ES3 = tracheostomy care *and* ventilator or respirator. ES2 = tracheostomy care *or* ventilator or respirator ES1 = infection *isolation*.

ADL scores are obtained by totaling the results from section G of the MDS, which describes a resident's bed mobility, eating, transfer, toileting, ambulation, and locomotion. The information for this section is obtained from the activities of daily living (ADL) tracker sheets that are completed by the certified nursing assistants every shift.

Category	ADL Score	RUG-IV
Rehabilitation Services		
Rehab ultra high + an extensive service	11–16	RUX
Rehab ultra high + an extensive service	2–10	RUL
Rehab very high + an extensive service	11–16	RVX
Rehab very high + an extensive service	2–10	RVL
Rehab high + an extensive service	11–16	RHX
Rehab high + an extensive service	2–10	RHL
Rehab medium + an extensive service	11–16	RMX
Rehab medium + an extensive service	2–10	RML
Rehab low + an extensive service	2–16	RLX
Note: there is no RLL		
Rehab ultra high	11–16	RUC
Rehab ultra high	6–10	RUB
Rehab ultra high	0–5	RUA
Rehab very high	11–16	RVC

Rehab very high	6–10	RVB
Rehab very high	0–5	RVA
Rehab high	11–16	RHC
Rehab high	6–10	RHB
Rehab high	0–5	RHA
Rehab medium	11–16	RMC
Rehab medium	6–10	RMB
Rehab medium	0–5	RMA
Note: there is no RLC		
Rehab low	11–16	RLB
Rehab low	0–10	RLA
Extensive Services		
Tracheostomy care *and* ventilator or respirator		ES3
Tracheostomy care *or* ventilator or respirator		ES2
Infection isolation		ES1
Special Care High		
1. Comatose and total ADL dependent	15–16 + depression	HE2
2. Septicemia	15–16	HE1
3. Diabetes	11–14 + depression	HD2
—daily injections (for 7 days)	11–14	HD1
—Insulin order changes on 2+ days		
4. Quadriplegia and ADL of 5 or more	6–10 + depression	HC2
5. COPD and SOB when lying flat	6–10	HC1
6. Fever with one of the following:	2–5 + depression	HB2
a). pneumonia	2–5	HB1
b). weight loss		
c). vomiting		
d). feeding tube with intake requirement		
7. Parenteral/IV feedings		
8. Respiratory therapy for 7 days (nebulizer)		
Special Care Low		

1. Cerebral palsy and ADLS of 5 or greater 2. Multiple sclerosis and ADLS of 5 or greater 3. Parkinson's disease and ADL of 5 or greater 4. Respiratory failure and oxygen 5. Feeding tube 6. Two stage 2 pressure ulcers with two treatments 7. Stage 3 or 4 pressure ulcer with ulcer treatments 8. Two or more venous/arterial ulcers with treatments 9. One stage 2 pressure ulcer and one venous/arterial ulcer with separate treatments		
	15–16 + depression	LE2
	15–16	LE1
	11–14 + depression	LD2
	11–14	LD1
	6–10 + depression	LC2
	6–10	LC1
	2–5 + depression	LB2
	2–5	LB1
Clinically Complex		
1. Residents with extensive services, special care high, or special care low who are highly functional with ADL score of 0–1 2. Pneumonia 3. Hemiplegia/hemiparesis and ADL of 5 or greater 4. Surgical wounds or open lesion with treatments 5. Burns 6. Chemotherapy while in the facility 7. Oxygen while in the facility 8. IV medications while in the facility 9. Transfusions while in the facility		
	15–16 + depression	CE2
	15–16	CE1
	11–14 + depression	CD2
	11–14	CD1
	6–10 + depression	CC2
	6–10	CC1
	2–5 + depression	CB2
	2–5	CB1
	0–1 + depression	CA2
	0–1	CA1
Behavior Symptoms and Cognitive Performance		

1. Cognitive impairment BIMS of 9 or less 2. Cognitive performance scale of 3 or less	2–5 + two or more restorative nursing	BB2
3. Hallucinations 4. Delusions	2–5 + two or less restorative nursing	BB1
5. Physical behavior symptoms toward others 6. Verbal behavior symptoms toward others	0–1 + two or more restorative nursing	BA2
7. Rejection of care 8. Wandering	0–1 + two or less restorative nursing	BA1
9. Restorative nursing services (toileting program; passive and/or active ROM; splint or brace assistance; bed mobility or walking training; transfer training; dressing and/or grooming training; eating and/or swallowing training; amputation/prosthesis care; communication training)		
Reduced Physical Function		
1. Behavioral symptoms and cognitive performance with ADL of 6–16 2. Residents who do not meet the conditions in any of the previous categories	15–16 + two or more restorative nursing	PE2
	15–16 + two or less restorative nursing	PE1
3. Restorative nursing services (toileting program; passive and/or active ROM; splint or brace assistance; bed mobility or walking training; transfer training; dressing and/or grooming training; eating and/or swallowing training; amputation/prosthesis care; communication training)	11–14 + two or more restorative nursing	PD2
	11–14 + two or less restorative nursing	PD1
	6–10 + two or more restorative nursing	PC2
	6–10 + two or less restorative nursing	PC1
	2–5 + two or more restorative nursing	PB2
	2–5 + two or less restorative nursing	PB1
	0–1 + two or more restorative nursing	PA2
	0–1 + two or less restorative nursing	PA1

MEDICAID SKILLED NURSING FACILITY CASE MIX (NEW YORK)

Case mix is a way for the nursing homes to receive revenues from the government for Medicaid and Medicaid-pending residents. It varies from state to state.

Case mix is done twice for the year in New York

1. The last Wednesday in April to the last Wednesday in July
2. The last Wednesday in October of one year through the last Wednesday in January of the following year

A thorough assessment must be done for each resident to determine if there is an existing skilled need or the necessity for same.

For recently admitted residents, IV hydration has a look back to hospital of seven days. Chemotherapy, radiation, transfusion, trache/ventilation, dialysis and oxygen usage have a look back period to the hospital of fourteen days.

Remember, everyone benefits from CMI. CMI provides needed funds from the government for resident care needs, staff hiring, and salary increases.

MEDICAID RUGS:

Category	ADL Score	RUG
Rehabilitation		
Rehab ultra high + an extensive service	16–18	RUX
Rehab ultra high + an extensive service	7–15	RUL
Rehab very high + an extensive service	16–18	RVX
Rehab very high + an extensive service	7–15	RVL
Rehab high + an extensive service	13–18	RHX
Rehab high + an extensive service	7–12	RHL

Rehab medium + an extensive service	15–18	RMX
Rehab medium + an extensive service	7–14	RML
Rehab low + an extensive service	7–18	RLX
Note: there is no RLL		
Rehab ultra high	16–18	RUC
Rehab ultra high	9–15	RUB
Rehab ultra high	4–8	RUA
Rehab very high	16–18	RVC
Rehab very high	9–15	RVB
Rehab very high	4–8	RVA
Rehab high	13–18	RHC
Rehab high	7–12	RHB
Rehab high	4–7	RHA
Rehab medium	15–18	RMC
Rehab medium	8–14	RMB
Rehab medium	4–7	RMA
Note: there is no RLC		
Rehab low	14–18	RLB
Rehab low	4–13	RLA
Extensive Services		

1. IV feedings in the last 7 days	7–18	SE3 (4–5 points)
2. IV medications in the last 14 days	7–18	
3. Suctioning in the last 14 days	7–18	SE2 (2–3 points)
4. Trache care in the last 14 days		
5. Vent or respirator care in the last 14 days		SE1 0–1 points)
This category works on a points system:		
1 point for a special care skill		
1 point for a clinical complex care skill		
1 point for impaired cognition		
1 point for IV medication		
1 point for IV feeding		
5 points maximum total can be obtained		
Special Care		
1. MS	17–18	SSC
2. Quadriplegic	15–16	SSB
3. Cerebral palsy with ADL greater than 9	7–14	SSA
4. Respiratory treatment for 7 consecutive days	0–7 falls in the clinically complex group	
5. Radiation		
6. Two or more stage 2 pressure ulcers with two or more treatments		
7. One or more stage 3 or 4 pressure ulcer with treatment		
8. Surgical wound		
9. Open lesion (cancerous)		
10. Tube feed with diagnosis of aphasia		
11. Fever with		
—dehydration		
—pneumonia		
—vomiting		
—weight loss		
Extensive Services with an ADL of 7 is an SSA		
Clinically Complex	17–18 + depression	CC2

1. Pneumonia	17–18	CC1
2. Foot wounds	12–16 + depression	CB2
3. Internal bleeding	12–16	CB1
4. Dehydration		
5. Tube feeding	4–11 + depression	CA2
6. Burns	4–11	CA1
7. Coma		
8. Sepsis		
9. Transfusion		
10. Oxygen		
11. Chemotherapy		
12. Hemiparesis with ADL greater than 9		
13. Dialysis		
14. Two MD visits and two MD orders in the last 14 days		
Impaired Cognition		
1. Score on MDS cognitive performance scale of greater than or equal to 3	6–10 + 2 nursing rehab	IB2
2. Nursing rehab are passive or active ROM, amputation care, splint care	6–10	IB1
3. Training in dressing, grooming, eating or swallowing, transferring, bed mobility or walking, communication, scheduled toileting program, or bladder retraining	4–5 + 2 nursing rehab	IA2
	4–5	IA1
Behavior Only		
	6–10 + 2 nursing rehab	BB2
Four or more documented days/week of wandering, verbal abuse, inappropriate behavior or resists care, hallucinations or delusions	6–10	BB1
	4–5 + 2 nursing rehab	BA2
	4–5	BA1
Physical Function Reduced		
	16–18 + 2 nursing rehab	PE2
There are no clinical conditions captured or maximized.	16–18	PE1
This section is based solely on the ADL score.	11–15 + 2 nursing rehab	PD2
	11–15	PD1

	9–10 + 2 nursing rehab	PC2
	9–10	PC1
	6–8 + 2 nursing rehab	PB2
	6–8	PB1
	4–5 + 2 nursing rehab	PA2
	4–5	PA1

NURSING MANAGEMENT/LEADERSHIP:

There are two old adages that still hold true: "You win more with honey than with lemons" and "Respect earns respect." OR "Respect is reciprocal"

What is your daily rapport with your staff? You will be amazed how much information staff will bring to your attention if they feel you will listen and not rush to conclusions or judgment.

Learn to say "Thank you for the work you do." Congratulate, appreciate, interact, and listen to your staff. Learn what is important to them.

Lead by example by showing your residents love, respect, and treat them with dignity. Be proficient at your job and always be willing to teach, not rebuke or discipline.

Be willing to help with tasks that you think are "beneath" you. When a unit is working short, the certified nursing assistants will never forget when you assist with two-person transfers or toileting. The nurses will never forget the day you did a few of the treatments or push the medication cart.

Give your staff credit when you learn something from them (e.g., the certified nursing assistant guiding you while you assist her during a Hoyer transfer, the nurse that has an efficient system for ensure the unit operates smoothly).

An effective manager at times wears the hat of a mother, father, counselor, or just a sounding board.

As much as possible, try to accommodate their requests for time off or change of schedule or some form of compromise.

NURSING DOCUMENTATION

A facility can provide top-notch care, but if it is not properly documented, it is as though it was never done! **If it is not documented, it is not done is the general slogan in this profession!**

An assessment cannot be done by an LPN by scope of practice. Therefore, it is prudent that with *every* acute change in the facility, the RN supervisor on duty assess and writes a progress note along with the LPN's note. This includes but is not limited to accidents/incidents, skin breaks, changes in resident's baseline, transfers and admissions. **Failure to comply with this may result in a citation in the area of scope and of practice!**

NOTE: If an acute condition leads to legal ramifications, the RN will be called into question as to whether the resident was properly assessed!

All acute changes require the doctor's documentation. It is important for nurses to know that after calling the doctor about an acute condition, it should be written in the doctor's communication book as a reminder to him/her to write a follow-up note.

If nurses are documenting issues that impact on other departments, they must make sure that the other department is aware so they can follow through.

As previously mentioned, for facilities with electronic medical records, morning meeting review of all progress notes written by all disciplines the previous day is an excellent way of monitoring the quality documentation in the facility and ensuring follow-up.

Facilities using paper records are advised to use the twenty-four-hour nursing report as a guide to review what is documented there with what is in the resident's chart.

When necessary, call nurses are called in to write clarification or late-entry notes.

Nursing notes must be clear, legible, concise and precise.

Nurses should always remember, five years from now, when they don't remember who a resident is and the circumstances surrounding a situation, their note should be able to stand on its own in a court of law.

NOTE: Nursing notes must not be ambiguous, i.e. notes must NOT be capable of double interpretation!

SBAR progress notes are an excellent way to keep the focus on accurate documentation.

Encourage oncoming or current nurse to always read the note of the outgoing or the previous nurse before to ensure that the focus of previous documentation is maintained.

For areas of documentation that require interdisciplinary documentation (e.g., weights, restraint reduction, accidents/incidents), have schedules in place to ensure these meetings take place and documentation is completed.

Whenever a nurse documents ANY issue in a resident's medical record it should be carried on the twenty four hour nursing report so that the next nurse is aware.

DEATH AND BURIAL ARRANGEMENTS

Social services play an integral role from pre-admission until discharge or death of a resident.

Upon admission and until discharge, the resident and family/legal representative must be made aware of any changes to the Resident's health, goals or discharge plans. While it is the responsibility of the doctor and or the nursing staff to notify the family of any changes in the Resident's health, the social worker plays an integral part in validating family notification.

Social services should be very proactive with discussing advance directives with families, especially DNR (do not resuscitate). For the sick and elderly, a DNR can help ensure death with dignity!

Death, even when it is inevitable, is often an unpleasant emotional experience. The death of a resident often leaves the remaining spouse and family with a sense of loss, a need to reach out and share or requiring direction to the next step. Even the most well prepared family at times appears ill-prepared in the event of death. It is the role of the medical or nursing team to notify families of a resident's death. However, social services should place a follow-up call and avail themselves to the family/legal representative to provide emotional support and offer guidance if needed.

In many instances, there are residents with no involved families or legal representative. The demise of these residents often prove a challenge for any facility.

Social Services must be proactive in discussing affordable burial plans with residents and families/legal representatives. In the demented or confused resident with no family/legal representative contact, every attempt should be made to make affordable burial arrangements prior to their demise.

NOTE: The list of residents with burial arrangements must be shared with nursing staff in the event of a death on the off-shift.

CASE STUDY

Resident is a 73 year old female with dementia, HTN, s/p CVA and colon cancer. Resident is incontinent of bowel and bladder and being cared for by family at home. Because of the family member's feeling of been the "sandwich generation" because of caring for a sick elderly parent and caring for young children, this led to caregiver burn out. Resident was hospitalized due to acute illness and subsequently placed in a long term care facility. During hospitalization for four days, family arrived at the hospital to visit resident and was informed by the resident that she fell and struck her head the night before and "they picked me up". As the primary contact listed on the resident's demographic sheet, family was never contacted about same. When nurse on duty who was doing a double was asked about the incident, she denied resident fell. However, when confronted with a hematoma on back of resident's head she stated oh yes she fell and we picked her up. I forgot about that. Resident struck her head in the fall and no neuro-checks or CAT scan was done. Resident was subsequently transferred to a long term care facility. Family went to visit about 4pm on a Saturday afternoon and saw resident seated in a wheelchair in the unit dining room with a seatbelt restraining her, her head on the table and the TV playing. The family was never contacted about a seatbelt and never gave consent for same. Resident asked family to put her to bed as she was tired. When nurse was asked if resident can be put to bed she stated resident is a high risk for fall. However, upon entering resident's room, family noted resident have appropriate fall interventions. Resident had a low position bed with a floor mat and an alarm! Why couldn't she be put to bed for comfort? Family requested an AMA (against medical advice) form and signed out resident and took her home even though she knew caring for her would be impossible. Within a few days, resident was in the hospital and subsequently admitted to a different long term care facility. Family arrived to visit resident and she was wearing her roommate's glasses. Resident had several children with no advance directives in place so instructions on her care to staff were often conflicting as children had different views on her care. Resident's condition deteriorated and she became unresponsive and was transferred back to the hospital. Family arrived at hospital one afternoon and observed a nursing instructor with five nursing students at resident's bedside. One student was practicing a subcutaneous injection on the resident. Hospital is a teaching hospital. At no time was family contacted to give consent for students to "practice" on resident. Family demanded that they all leave the room promptly. Family cried and said to the the 'unresponsive' resident "go on home to your God, your children and grandchildren will be okay." Tears rolled down the checks of the 'unresponsive' resident. Four hours later, family received a call from hospital that resident passed away peacefully in her sleep.

How many errors were made in this case study?

This is a true story and that resident was my mother!

BIBLIOGRAPHY

- The Long Term Care Survey, October 2010 Edition. Published by American Health Care Association
- Long Term E-Newsletter 2/27/15 Edition on 5 Star rating
- New York State Department of Health Bureau of Long Term Services—Facility Survey Report (FSR)—DOH 1550 (7/95)
- NEW YORK State Medicaid SNF Case-Mix
- Rapid Rug-IV Guide
- INTERACT 4.0 tool
- SBAR Communication Form by INTERACT
- STOP and WATCH Early Warning Tool
- Department of Health and Human Services Centers for Medicare & Medicaid Services-Entrance Conference Worksheet. Form CMS 20045 (11/2010)
- Scope and Severity Matrix. Freed Maxick & Bataglia, PC
- New York State Department of Health Division of Residential Services-Nursing Home Incident Reporting Manual. General Information (NH DAL 11-12; Incident Reporting System)
- Centers for Medicare and Medicaid Services. 2012. Resident Assessment Instrument Comprehensive User Manual. Version 3.0
- www.Medicare.gov Nursing Home Compare/About/Ratings. Html
- Medicare.gov--The Official US Government Site for Medicare
- Centers for Medicare and Medicaid Services Official Site www.cms.gov
- The Lippincott Manual of Nursing Practices (7th Edition) Philadelphia. Lippincott, Williams & Wilkins.
- Heaton Manual
- MCN Healthcare Home Health Policy & Procedure Manual
- Center for Disease Control and Prevention 24/7 Saving Lives and Protecting people. www.cdc.gov
- Centers for Medicare and Medicaid Services, Publication #100-07, State Operations Manual.

- Centers for Medicare and Medicaid Services 2010 Edition Long Term Care Survey
- The American Society of Consultant Pharmacists (ASCP) www.ascp.com
- US Department of Health and Human Services (DHHS), Food and Drug Administration (FDAP) www.fda.gv/cder
- National Food Safety Information Network's Gateway to Government Food Safety Information at www.FoodSafety.gov
- American Medical Directors Association at "www.amda.com

INDEX

A

abuse, 2-3, 8, 10, 20, 27, 50, 58, 60, 62-63, 66-70, 73, 76, 96, 107, 119
accountability record, 151
ADL, 155-56, 179, 185-88, 191-92
admissions, 22, 30, 90, 173-74, 181-82
  new, 175, 182
affected site, 28, 33
amputation/prosthesis care, 188
antidepressant, 42-43
appetite, 20, 42-43, 99, 103
appointment, 140-41
areas, visible, 11
assessment
  pressure ulcer risk, 28
  quarterly, 17-18

B

bed mobility, 185, 188, 192
blood, 115-16, 130, 142-43
bowel movement, 181-82
brace assistance, 188

C

case mix, 189
catheters, 119-20
  permanent, 119
change schedule, 118-19
chemotherapy, 82, 187, 189, 192
closets, 94, 159, 165

cognitive performance, 187-88
collage, 65
communication training, 188
community, xi, xiii, 5, 27, 89-90, 155, 181-82
Comprehensive Assessment, 17-18, 46, 55, 63, 66, 81, 97, 102, 109, 112, 114, 117, 120, 123, 129
conditions, acute, 30, 100, 181, 195
consultants, xv, 4, 87, 140-41, 144, 147, 150
consults, 100, 140-41, 144, 147, 149-50

D

dehydration, 111, 113-14, 164, 191-92
department heads, 96, 171, 173-75
depression, 42-43, 46, 100, 186-87, 191-92
devices, 27, 30-31, 34, 79, 126, 130, 146-47, 151-53
diagnosis, 5, 16, 19, 33, 43, 90, 108, 114, 122, 131-32, 135, 140, 182, 191
dialysis, 9, 86, 101, 113, 115-17, 189, 192
dietitian, xv, 29, 34, 72, 99-100, 103, 113-14, 117
discharges, 11, 13, 16, 52, 60, 89-92, 173, 197
discrepancies, 44, 149-50, 175
doctors, 20, 28, 150
document, 10, 21, 43, 150

JANE GABBIDON

treatments, 9-10, 28-29, 31-34, 42, 46,
      82, 92, 108, 115, 122, 126, 128,
      140-41, 187, 191
Tylenol, 21-22, 29, 149

U

ulcers, venous/arterial, 187
units, 40, 50, 54, 58-59, 65, 72, 90, 95,
      105, 134-35, 157, 160, 163, 193

V

ventilator, 185-86

W

wanderers, 64-66
water, 101, 159-60, 162, 165, 174
weight fluctuations, 117
weight loss, 44, 82, 101-2, 181, 186, 191
wounds, 18, 26-31, 86, 135